How to get pregnant

How to get pregnant

The Zhai Programme

for successful conception

Dr Xiao-Ping Zhai

hamlyn

In loving memory of my mother.
Without her I would not be where I am today.

An Hachette UK Company
www.hachette.co.uk

First published in Great Britain in 2012 by Hamlyn,
a division of Octopus Publishing Group Ltd, Endeavour House,
189 Shaftesbury Avenue, London WC2H 8JY
www.octopusbooks.co.uk
www.octopusbooksusa.com

Distributed in the US by Hachette Book Group USA,
237 Park Avenue, New York, NY 10017, USA

Distributed in Canada by Canadian Manda Group,
165 Dufferin Street, Toronto, Ontario, Canada M6K 3H6

ISBN 978 0 600 62192 8

A CIP catalogue record for this book is available from the British Library.

Printed and bound by CPI Group (UK) Ltd, Croydon, CR0 4YY.

10 9 8 7 6 5 4 3 2 1

Warning Do not take Chinese herbs without first consulting a qualified Traditional
Chinese Medicine (TCM) practitioner. A list of TCM practitioners can be found on the
Association of Traditional Chinese Medicine website, at *www.atcm.co.uk*. All members
of the ATCM hold a university, college or other recognized professional qualification
and are bound by the Association's Code of Ethics and Code of Practice at all times.

TCM and acupuncture are powerful. They have been proven to be very effective in the
treatment of many conditions and have been safely practised for centuries in China,
but would be harmful if administered by an inadequately trained person. Therefore,
it is essential that only properly qualified practitioners should prescribe Chinese
herbal medication or use acupuncture. It takes several years of specialized study to
understand the theories and principles of TCM and to be proficient in the practice of
Chinese herbal medicine and acupuncture.

CONTENTS

Foreword

We have many patients who are trying to have a baby who express an interest in Traditional Chinese Medicine with Acupuncture. The lack of regulation and oversight in this area had always given us cause for concern. It was therefore a real delight and pleasure to find in Dr Zhai a physician who both understood the scientific rigour and evidence base of Western medicine but at the same time was able to introduce our patients to an alternative approach and philosophy encompassing Traditional Chinese Medicine.

Our patients find reassurance in her holistic view of fertility treatment, and genuinely appreciate her honesty and candour. Over the years we have shared the care of many couples who having been trying to start a family for a long time. These couples have often undergone multiple unsuccessful attempts at IVF and are looking for a fresh approach that offers them hope and inspiration. The Zhai Clinic is able to offer all these things and deliver results.

There are many practitioners of TCM in Harley Street, but what makes Dr Zhai unique is that she is able to focus on the individual needs of her patients and advise them on the best of what conventional Western medicine and TCM can offer. She is able to find that right balance between realistic expectation and the hope that will sustain couples through treatment.

Mr Stuart Lavery MRCOG
Consultant Gynaecologist and Director IVF Hammersmith,
Hammersmith Hospital

Introducing the Zhai Programme

Having a baby should be the most natural thing in the world but, sadly, it is not always the simplest. Sometimes, when you decide you are ready to start a family, you discover that your wishes don't go according to plan.

As you have picked up this book I imagine that you are one of those people for whom pregnancy hasn't happened; that you are looking for answers and entering the minefield of fertility information, trying to understand how to take control of your body and choose the right path.

In the Western fertility world there is an ongoing debate as to whether assisted fertility treatment should be the first resort; or whether relaxation, nutrition, supplements, exercise and a healthy lifestyle can improve the chances of pregnancy naturally. There is a big gap between the two camps.

In all instances, the key to a successful pregnancy is reproductive health: a healthy egg and a healthy sperm merge to become a healthy embryo. For implantation to take place, a healthy blood supply is needed within the woman's reproductive system, especially to the uterus (womb). This is the case whether conception occurs naturally or with the help of assisted fertility treatment.

Assisted conception is a magnificent tool for overcoming many infertility conditions; the advancements made over the years have transformed the chances of a woman conceiving. However, *no* assisted fertility treatment can improve the *quality* of the egg or sperm; medical doctors can only select the healthiest from what the man and woman are able to produce. That is why my own belief is that the initial focus should be on improving the normal function of the reproductive system, to ensure that the body is functioning well enough to be able to conceive and maintain a pregnancy *before* subjecting the body to the rigours of assisted fertility treatment, such as Intra-Uterine Insemination (IUI), In-Vitro Fertilization (IVF) or Intra-Cytoplasmic Sperm Injection (ICSI).

East meets West

Traditional Chinese Medicine (TCM) is a form of medicine that has been used in China and Asia for thousands of years to successfully treat millions of people. It is still widely used today, alongside Western medicine, as a primary choice of treatment. I have written this book because I believe that through the use of TCM, both women and men can improve reproductive health and their chances of conceiving, whether naturally or when using assisted conception. I am not claiming that TCM is a better treatment than the Western alternative, but in my experience the best results are achieved when doctors of both disciplines work together to diagnose and treat infertility problems.

My early career

Before we go any further, let me explain how I have reached this point in my medical career. I studied Western medicine in China, graduating in 1980. The first two years of my junior doctor's career were full of inspiration. I was like a sponge, desperate to absorb knowledge and experience and to put into practice what I had learnt so that I could help those who were in need.

During the course of my work I often found that patients whose problems were associated with diseases such as diabetes, asthma, or with persistent coughs were not being cured, no matter how many antibiotics or steroids they were taking. They would ask me instead for repeat prescriptions of Chinese medicine that they had been given by their TCM doctors.

I felt there was a big gap between just treating the acute symptoms of the disease, and restoring the general health and wellbeing of the body, necessary to recover from disease. So many instances of acute disease become chronic as the human body struggles to return to normal functioning after surgery or persistent treatment with drugs such as antibiotics.

TCM doesn't replace the need for medicines and surgery but it can certainly play an important role in restoring the normal functioning of the human body, essential for fighting disease and healing the body. I noticed that patients who managed their chronic health problems with TCM showed a remarkable improvement, which inspired me to study TCM professionally. At that time the Chinese government encouraged doctors of Western medicine to study Chinese medicine too, so for nearly six years I treated my patients during the day and studied TCM in the evenings and at weekends. I gained my qualification as a Doctor of TCM in 1985, and thereafter was able to use both Western and Chinese medicine at the same time, although I didn't specialize in fertility straight away.

My interest in fertility

I later moved to London and started a general practice. My very first infertile couple came to see me in 1995. They both were in their early 40s, and for seven years they had been undergoing all the conventional investigations and treatments. They were diagnosed as having 'unexplained infertility'. They had failed five IVF cycles and were told there was nothing more that could be done. However, after four months of TCM treatment they conceived and gave birth to a healthy little girl. This wonderful result astonished me as much as it did the couple. I began investigating what treatment options were available for infertile couples in this country and how successful the treatments were.

During my research I found that many infertile couples had been offered semen analysis, hormone tests, tubal patency tests, ultrasound scans or even laparoscopy when necessary, as well as ovulation induction using drugs such as Clomiphene, followed by the assisted fertility options of IUI, IVF or ICSI. There was, however, nothing that investigated whether the body was fit for reproduction.

One gynaecologist I spoke to was adamant that, 'there is no way your TCM can stand a chance in the West, as IVF success rates are so high [around 20 per cent at that time], and it is so quick to get a woman pregnant. ICSI takes just one needle to inject the sperm into an egg. It's very simple and easy, whereas TCM takes too long. No one would be interested in it.'

But another gynaecologist, at one of the most respected London hospitals, had a totally different opinion. He said, 'That's rubbish. IVF is too invasive, with a low success rate.' He agreed that it would be good if there were methods for helping infertile couples other than just IVF. He was interested in TCM and applied for research funding for a trial to investigate its effectiveness. He failed to get a grant, so I decided to go ahead with my treatments anyway. Since then, I have specialized in fertility treatment.

The Zhai Clinic
I founded The Zhai Clinic in 1993, and opened my clinic on Harley Street in London, in 1996. I am pleased to say that our success rate has been at a consistently high level.

Since that time I have seen many, many patients who always ask me the same question: *'We have a very good lifestyle, we don't smoke, we drink very little, neither of us is overweight, we have been taking all the supplements advised for a few years but we still can't conceive. Why not?'*

Those who are undergoing assisted conception will often add, *'We have always produced embryos during the IVF/ICSI process but the embryo doesn't last. The implantation is the problem.'*

Of the 869 female patients who completed our recommended TCM treatment programme from 1995 to 2008, 78 per cent became pregnant. The average age was 37.8 years, each of these women had, on average, been trying to conceive for 3.8 years and failed, and had undergone an average of four cycles of assisted fertility treatment. Yet few had been offered any investigation into why they weren't conceiving or any other treatment apart from assisted fertility treatments such IVF or ICSI.

The key to success
I believe that our success rate is so high because most patients who have trouble conceiving are *not* suffering from mechanical problems such as blocked fallopian tubes (these can be fixed by surgery or bypassed using IVF). The most common causes of IVF failure are poor sperm production, poor-quality eggs, malfunction of the ovaries or the blood supply within the abdomen not being healthy enough. Couples

who find it difficult to conceive have problems that can often be helped by kick-starting the reproductive system, improving sperm quantity and quality, and improving the menstrual cycle, the functioning of the ovaries and the quality of the eggs. To achieve this, I use Traditional Chinese Medicine.

At The Zhai Clinic we use a combination of Chinese herbs, acupuncture and healthy lifestyle advice to help our patients. We monitor progress closely in order to fully understand the body of each individual and to give them the treatments they need to achieve optimum fertility and reproductive health.

The aim of this book

Trying, and failing, to conceive can cause emotional distress and put pressure on relationships, so I hope this book helps you to understand how much can be done to improve your chances of getting pregnant. My intention is to arm you with as much information as possible so that you can make choices about how to prepare yourself for a successful pregnancy, and about the way you would like to conceive, whether you are undergoing IVF treatment or trying to conceive naturally.

Many patients have told me that I perform miracles, which is wonderful feedback, but that is not how I see it. My work is all about understanding how the human body works naturally, assessing what needs to be done to improve its health and, by encouraging patients to follow the TCM advice, to hopefully optimize their chances of one day holding their own baby son or daughter in their arms.

TCM isn't a quick fix, it requires patience to allow your body to change and improve. Sometimes this involves changing your entire lifestyle – what you eat, drink and how you exercise. But it's a system that has been tried and tested for thousands of years and I have reason to believe in it completely. So do the hundreds of women I have treated who have gone on to have babies using TCM.

Dr Xiao-Ping Zhai
January 2012

PART 1

INTRODUCING TRADITIONAL CHINESE MEDICINE

Chapter 1

THE PRINCIPLES OF TRADITIONAL CHINESE MEDICINE

This book has been written to help you decide if Traditional Chinese Medicine (TCM) might help you, whether you have just decided to start trying for a baby or you are experiencing fertility problems. As you read I shall introduce you to my personalized treatment programme, which marries modern science with ancient Chinese medicine. I make use of the best of both Eastern and Western medicine. The main difference between the two is that TCM treats the whole body, rather than individual parts or symptoms.

You may be familiar with the Western medical terms I use but you may be very unfamiliar with TCM and the role it can play in fertility. I will try to explain the language in a way that is accessible and familiar. You may be aware of the more popular aspects of TCM – perhaps you've had acupuncture, or know someone who has; perhaps you've walked past a clinic or shop with shelves stacked with dried roots and other unfamiliar herbs; or perhaps you've read about treatments in the health pages of newspapers or on the Internet. But to understand fully what TCM is you need to appreciate how deeply rooted and well established it is in Eastern culture, and how it differs from, but works alongside, Western medicine.

TCM treats the body as an integrated system and recognizes that energy levels can get out of balance, or organ function can underachieve or be overactive.

TCM comprises mainly acupuncture and herbal medicine. Acupuncture involves the insertion of fine needles into different parts of the body to stimulate the human body network to balance and function properly. Herbal medicine has powerful healing properties which work on the internal organs and reproductive system. It aims to clear obstruction, rectifies the balance between *yin* and *yang* in the organs (as I will explain) and helps to restore normal bodily functions. Most importantly, herbs have proved capable of reducing chromosomal abnormality in male sperm and female eggs, so improving sperm and egg quality.

TCM is a unique, distinct and independent medical system that has been practised in China for more than 5,000 years, long before Western medicine began. It has developed over the centuries, supported by a wealth of clinical experience and deep understanding of the human body and how it works. In Western societies it is often called alternative or complementary medicine but, for millions of people in China and other Asian countries, TCM is still a primary method of healthcare, although Western medicine is now usually practised in parallel. For me it is not either/or; it is about taking an integrated approach.

The ancient method involves sophisticated medical diagnosis. It uses a combination of herbs, acupuncture, massage (*tui na*) and diet to diagnose physical ailments and prevent or treat diseases. It has never lost its popularity or its authority, partly because it has been proven to work. Over thousands of years, millions of people can testify to it.

TCM is particularly effective in fertility healthcare because it has few or no side effects, improves the overall health of the patient and produces high clinical pregnancy rates.

In this book I hope to help you increase your chances of pregnancy by improving your body's overall health, reducing the need for assisted intervention, or boosting your chances of success when assisted intervention is necessary.

THE HISTORY OF TCM

2700 BC

The earliest recorded mention of TCM dates back to around 2700 BC in the *Huang Di Nei Jing*, the Yellow Emperor's classic volume of internal medicine. This is the earliest source outlining the theories of *yin* and *yang* and the five elements that form the basis of TCM. The work makes many references to female anatomy and to the diagnosis and treatment of gynaecological problems. Although the book was credited to the enlightened Yellow Emperor, who presided over a time of great scientific and social advances, it was probably written by several authors over an extended period of time. Revisions were made up until AD 25.

500 BC

One of the most famous and revered of the ancient physicians, Bian Que, used pulse-taking and acupuncture as the basis for his renowned medical diagnostic technique. He achieved almost godlike status when he attended the Queen of Hu, who was said to have died, and used his diagnostic techniques to seemingly bring her back to life. He is said to have influenced many physicians of the time through his work, *Bian Que Nei Jing*, though no copy of it survives.

221 BC–AD 220

Two other classic medical books were written during the Qin and Han Dynasties of 221 BC–AD 220. Shen Nong is an historical (and some say mythological) figure, who is known as 'the divine farmer'. The *Classic of Herbal Medicine*, which carries his name, lists some 365 Chinese medicines and outlines some of the principles by which herbal concoctions were made to cure imbalances. During this era Chinese medicine was becoming more formalized and Zhang Zhongjing's *Treatise on Cold-Induced and Miscellaneous Diseases* established the use of diagnosis based on overall analysis of signs and symptoms with its prescriptions forming the basis of modern clinical practice.

Chinese Middle Ages

During this period, the theory of pulse diagnosis was written down and the first complete reference guide to acupuncture was compiled. During the early Qing Dynasty, in the 15th and 16th centuries, many gynaecological books were written, mainly on the origin and treatment of gynaecological diseases. Several of the formulas relating to the regulation of the menstrual cycle and the importance of Kidney essence also date back to this time.

17th and 18th centuries

The West came into contact with Chinese medicine during the 17th century when it was first introduced by the Jesuits, who brought information back from China. The eminent English physician Sir John Floyer (1694–1734) was so impressed with an ancient Chinese text on pulse-taking that he undertook a study of the subject himself: the earliest study of its kind on Chinese medicine in the West. He published two books on the diagnostic powers of pulse-taking.

19th and 20th centuries

Acupuncture became established in the West around 1821, when J M Churchill FRCS published the first official account of the use of acupuncture in Britain.

The introduction of Western medicine to China began during the 19th century when Western doctors travelled there. They regarded the traditional methods with distrust. The power of Western thought infiltrated up to the level of high office and in 1929 the Chinese government tried to abandon TCM altogether. But the people resisted as it was too well established and worked as a proven diagnostic and treatment method. During the Cultural Revolution (1966–76) the traditional methods were again encouraged and now the two systems coexist harmoniously in China.

The use of TCM has progressed slowly in the West, although in the 1960s and 1970s Eastern spiritual philosophy became fashionable and attracted a much wider audience to the therapeutic benefits of yoga, meditation, Tai Chi and TCM.

21st century

Twenty-first century modernization has its roots in the era of Chairman Mao, who actively encouraged Western doctors to study Chinese medicine and also wanted students of Chinese medicine to study the Western approach to anatomy and physiology. As a result, a more integrated approach continues to evolve. TCM remedies are now commonly available in pill form and are becoming subject to greater regulation.

In the West there is an increase in the number of universities and other institutions offering degree courses in TCM. There are now over 1,000 TCM practitioners in the UK alone and well over 6,000 acupuncturists. After so many thousands of years, the best of East and West is beginning to merge.

TCM history may help us understand the system of medicine that I'm writing about in this book, which requires a different approach and understanding of the human body to Western ideas. It is a skilled discipline that has been studied and refined by some of the most respected and advanced minds over centuries. TCM is a vital holistic system of health and healing, based on the notion of harmony and balance, and employs the concepts of moderation and prevention. It has been used consistently, and successfully, no matter who has been in power and irrespective of the development of other ideologies and influences.

An integrated approach

Before we look at how Chinese medicine works with the human body I feel it's important to stress that when you consult a TCM practitioner you benefit from the wisdom of both TCM *and* Western medicine. This is because, from the 16th century onwards, TCM integrated aspects of Western medicine into its teachings. Consulting a TCM practitioner isn't a question of turning your back on any advances in Western medicine or rejecting any Western advice because your TCM doctor will undoubtedly use a combination of both traditions. The aim will be to look at ways to help your body improve its own fertility levels – and also to improve your chances of success with IVF or other assisted methods of conception.

As I trained first in Western medicine I am hugely grateful for the benefits it has brought, particularly in the areas of fertility treatment. The valuable techniques and monitoring methods allow us to investigate and see inside the body; to measure and monitor hormone levels; and to evaluate sperm counts – all of which are important aspects of uncovering why a couple is unable to conceive.

Western fertility treatments can bypass physical problems, such as blocked fallopian tubes, for example, by introducing a single sperm to an egg that has been mechanically harvested. It also allows us to use embryo screening (using pre-implantation genetic diagnosis, or PGD) to look at the genetic make-up of a single egg or embryo; to evaluate its potential for developing into a pregnancy and place in the womb only those that are free of genetic abnormalities. However, these treatments are invasive and emotionally and physically draining. They also have a low success rate. So the question we must ask is, *'Why, even if a woman's egg is fertilized outside the body by a sperm, are so few embryos successfully implanted to produce a healthy baby?'*

I believe that our own bodies can tell us the answer. My approach is to look for signals that the body gives out and to interpret them, to understand why the body isn't conceiving. Chinese medicine offers the chance to improve the health of the egg or sperm and the uterus, and discover where the problems lie *before* undergoing the emotional and physical stresses of attempting to get pregnant or opting for assisted fertility treatment.

As I always explain to my patients, the decision to use TCM is like deciding how to travel to work. Some people may walk, others may go by car, bus, train, taxi or even helicopter. It's good to have a choice, but the choice should always suit your individual needs. If you could drive home in just ten minutes, why would you choose to fly by helicopter when it's unnecessary, expensive and you will become stressed when trying to find a place to land? Choosing to use TCM is like taking the most comfortable option for travel. It works *for* you, not against you. For example:

- When a man and woman who are failing to conceive come to my clinic we look at how regular the woman's menstrual cycle is, consider whether her periods are light or heavy, whether they are clotty or not; whether she suffers pain and, if so, does that pain need easing with painkillers?
- If a woman has tried IVF or ICSI and has successfully produced many eggs, or even had some embryos develop but fail to implant, we look not only at the number of the follicles produced but also at what size they are on the day of the egg collection, to identify whether most of the follicles are immature or whether she simply has a poor response.
- We look at why a man's sperm count or sperm motility (how well it 'swims') is low or why there is a high level of abnormal sperm.
- We look at why the woman's womb cannot maintain a pregnancy and work with her body to promote its function, to make it more productive and create the optimum conditions for a pregnancy to thrive.

Lifestyle factors such as drinking, smoking, a poor diet eaten on the run and sometimes even too much intense exercise can all tip the body out of balance. This isn't just a Chinese belief; Western medicine also recognizes the need for homeostasis – the body's ability to internally adjust and rebalance its biochemistry so that enzymes and hormones are released at the correct levels.

The difference lies in the approach to treatment. Western medicine tends to focus on eliminating symptoms through the use of medication, whereas TCM uses the symptoms to understand what is happening within the organs of the body. For example, many patients go to their doctor complaining of 'feeling low or anxious'. A Western doctor might prescribe antidepressants, recommend time off work or suggest blood tests to look at iron or thyroid levels. In Chinese medicine, as well as looking at iron or thyroid levels, we also focus on internal organ function to assess the vital energy levels. It is the balance of this energy we shall look at now.

The theory of *yin* and *yang*

The key to health in TCM is achieving and maintaining balance, especially the balance of 'essential energies' that flow through the body and are responsible for the harmonious working of the interrelated essential organs. In particular, TCM seeks to balance *yin* and *yang* energies.

Yin and *yang* are two opposite and complementary types of energy, thought to be present in the universe and within the human body. *Yin* and *yang* describe the interdependent relationship of opposing but complementary forces believed to be necessary for a healthy life. The *yin-yang* theory provides the rationale for the practice of TCM. The goal is to maintain a balance of *yin* and *yang* in all things.

Each energy, while balancing the other, also has a trace of the other within itself – as symbolized by the contrasting dot within each section of the *yin-yang* symbol. So, although *yin* (the white part of the symbol) might be described as a more 'feminine'

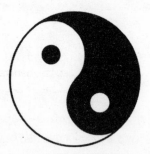

energy, women also have *yang* (the black part of the symbol) or 'masculine' energy within them – and vice versa for men. Each energy should ideally hold the force of the other in check and in balance, so neither energy overpowers the other. When imbalance does occur, there will be an 'excess' of *yin* or *yang*, which in turn will deplete the level of the opposite energy and make it 'deficient'.

The *yin-yang* principle can be seen in all aspects of the physical and spiritual world. For example:

Yin symbolizes: Night, cold, dark, moon, rest, earth, feminine, internal, back, below. It symbolizes bodily functions related to nourishment, moisture and cooling. It is associated with passivity, sleep, calmness and intuition.

Yang symbolizes: Day, heat, light, sun, activity, heaven, masculine, external, front, above. It also symbolizes bodily functions related to movement, transformation and heat, and is associated with mental and physical activity and emotions such as anger and laughter.

But within the human body, as in nature, the balance between *yin* and *yang* isn't fixed. It fluctuates throughout our lives and with each passing day; it can be influenced by what we eat or drink as well as how we act, what we think and how we feel. TCM sees the body as an integrated whole in which mind and emotions have a significant effect on our physiology.

In TCM, when we start treatment we classify the patient into a type (also known as a pattern or syndrome). We then seek to rectify overactive or underactive *yin* and *yang* in the internal organs, and rebalance whichever aspect is out of balance to restore the body to its normal functioning.

Vital energy: the nature of *qi*

Yin-yang also encompasses the body's metabolism and describes the balance between anabolic functions (that build up body tissue) and catabolic functions (that generate physical energy). Healthy physiology and metabolism depend on a steady supply of vital energy or *qi* (pronounced 'chi') that flows through the body.

Understanding the nature of *qi* is the cornerstone of understanding TCM and it is a concept that doesn't really exist in Western medicine. *Qi* energy serves to 'warm' the body, protecting it from external causes of disease, generating and distributing body fluids and blood. Each vital organ has its own *qi* for carrying out its special function.

The *qi* flows along set routes or pathways known as meridians (sometimes called channels), and it is these meridians that are mapped by acupuncturists when they insert needles to unblock the flow of *qi* or increase its power. There are 12 main meridians, each related to a specific organ (see pages 38–52).

- *Qi* that *motivates and warms* is classed as *yang* – and is energy related.
- *Qi* that *nourishes and moistens* is classed as *yin* – and is blood related.

Functions of *qi*
In every case, the basic functions of *qi* are:

- Protecting
- Warming
- Moving
- Transforming
- Holding
- Raising

For example, Spleen *qi* holds the blood in the blood vessels, while Liver *qi* ensures the smooth flow of *qi* throughout the whole body and in all directions. If one of these functions becomes impaired, *qi* 'disease' presents itself. Common examples are *qi* deficiency manifesting as tiredness, or *qi* stagnation (applying mostly to *qi* of the Liver) manifesting as premenstrual tension.

The role of *qi* in TCM

In TCM, *qi* is an invisible energy force that flows freely in a healthy person, but when it is weakened or blocked, a person becomes ill. Specifically, *the illness is a result of the blockage, rather than the blockage being the result of the illness*.

This holistic approach to medical diagnosis differs considerably from the Western approach, and so the treatment method is also quite different. Conventional Western medicine tends to remove blockages surgically or aims to prevent or cure symptoms by means of synthetic pharmaceuticals. In TCM it's believed that *qi* is the fundamental essence of the human body and that the movement and transformation of *qi* can explain all physiological behaviour. TCM works with the body and uses plants and roots to unblock or transform the *qi* so that the body disperses the symptoms. Traditionally, the herbs used were wild; nowadays, some are still wild and some are farm grown.

TYPES OF *QI*

Qi has been variously translated as 'energy' or 'life force', but within that there are various types of *qi*:

Ancestral *qi* (*yuan qi*) is inherited from our birth parents. There is a finite amount which, once depleted, cannot be regenerated. Its origin is in the Kidneys.

Postnatal *qi* (*hou tain qi*) originates in the Spleen. It is absorbed from the environment, via the air, water, food and other elements.

Defensive *qi* (*wei qi*) protects the exterior of the body.

Nutritive *qi* (*ying qi*) nourishes the interior of the body.

Each of the organs of the body also has its own *qi*.

QI AND BLOOD

In Chinese medicine, Blood is a very dense material form of *qi*, with *qi* infusing life into Blood. In terms of *yin* and *yang*, *qi* is *yang* and Blood is *yin*.

Blood is mostly derived from the *qi* stored in the Kidneys and from *qi* derived from ingested food and drink transformed by the Spleen. Thus, Blood and *qi* have a very close relationship, of which there are four aspects:

- *Qi* generates Blood, as *qi* is essential for the production of Blood. A deficiency of *qi* will eventually lead to a deficiency of Blood.
- *Qi* moves Blood, as *qi* is the motive force of Blood. So if *qi* stagnates it cannot move Blood, leading to Blood stasis.
- *Qi* holds Blood in the blood vessels, preventing haemorrhages.
- Blood nourishes *qi* and provides the basic material for *qi*.

In TCM it is said that, 'Qi *is the commander of Blood and Blood is the mother of* qi.'

Traditional Chinese Medicine recognizes three basic Blood disorders:

Deficiency of Blood That is, when not enough is produced (see page 109).

Blood stasis For example, due to internal haemorrhage caused by a trauma, or due to *qi* stagnation or Cold (see page 105).

Blood Heat is mostly due to Liver Heat. For example, as a result of long-term Liver *qi* stagnation due to emotional repression or innate constitution (see page 106).

An insufficient volume of Blood in the body, or Blood deficiency, can cause illness and diseases. This could result from excessive blood loss through childbirth, an operation or injury; or could be a malfunction of the digestive system, failing to absorb the fine essence from foods that transforms into Blood. It may also be the result of a failure to eliminate stagnant Blood and to produce new Blood.

BLOOD STASIS

This refers to impaired Blood circulation or the local accumulation of stagnant Blood. The main signs of Blood stasis in women who are having trouble conceiving are: endometriosis, ovarian cysts, painful periods with blood clots and a purple tongue and lips.

Understanding body balance

When *yin* and *yang* are out of balance, the problem is described as displaying either an *excess syndrome* or a *deficient syndrome*.

Excess syndrome

This occurs when there is overactivity in the body's organs, in the case of illness (especially an infection) or when there is a blockage of some kind so there may be pathogens present (bacteria or germs). Excess syndrome is treated with the **clearing or reducing method**, which is designed to reduce the impact of toxicity and overload on the body.

Deficient syndrome

This occurs when the body is lacking something – for example, the body may be *qi* deficient (lacking in energy or suffering from overuse). Deficient syndrome is treated with the **nourishing or tonifying method**, designed to build up the depleted functions of the body.

In TCM the aim is always to remove excess and replenish deficiency in order to maintain balance in the body. As we look at treating fertility problems with TCM, we'll see how an imbalance in *yin* and *yang* is involved in every aspect of the reproductive process, from the Western diagnosis, laboratory tests, menstrual cycles and sperm production to the successful implantation and maintenance of a healthy pregnancy. Where the Western treatment might induce ovulation to stimulate the reproductive system, Chinese medicine encourages the body to restore its own equilibrium.

The Three Treasures (*San bao*)

In the long-established Chinese tradition, the 'Three Treasures' are the essential components of life that make us human. These are:

Jing The basic constitution, nutritive essence, reproductive essence, seed.

Qi This can be described as energy. It forms the basis of all functional activity, is the foundation of *yin* and *yang* and a moving force. See pages 19–21.

Shen Individual personality, consciousness and spirit.

Jing, *qi* and *shen* are not separate entities; each influences the health and balance of the other. Their interaction affects vitality, mental stability, life and, of course, fertility.

When these vital substances are depleted, an imbalance is created which causes illness and promotes ageing.

The Three Treasures make up our constitution and represent an interaction between the body, mind and spirit. Although we cannot determine our basic constitution, we can positively affect our Three Treasures through the way we live our lives, thus maintaining balanced bodily functions and a harmonious mind.

THE PROPERTIES OF *JING, QI* AND *SHEN*

	Related organ	Fundamental property
JING	Kidneys	Constitution at birth
QI	Stomach/Spleen	Personal wellbeing
SHEN	Heart	Inner spirit

THE NATURE OF *JING*

Jing means 'essence'. It can be compared to our genetic make-up or basic constitution and is linked to the Kidneys. It is said to be inherited from our parents: a unique blend of energies formed at conception. *Jing* forms the basis for growth, reproduction and development, and nourishes the mind. Parents with strong *jing* will pass strong *jing* on to their children, unless there is unexpected trauma during the pregnancy. *Jing* is the basic essence formed in the embryo and the unborn baby during pregnancy and determines individual strength and vitality. Thus plentiful *jing* contributes to longevity and increases fertility as it influences the egg and sperm quality.

The quality and quantity of *jing* we have are fixed. We cannot increase *jing* but we can maintain it or restore it, through a balanced lifestyle and healthy diet. Any extreme behaviour or habits will invariably deplete *jing*.

THE IMPORTANCE OF *QI*

Qi is explained more fully on pages 19–21. It has various forms and functions in the body. It is the foundation of all the *yin* and *yang* in the body. It is reflected in the Stomach and Spleen (digestive system). *Qi* can be enhanced by acquiring further *qi* from the air we breathe and the nutrients we consume. *Qi* circulates in the meridians of the body (see pages 38–52) and is the force behind all the functional activity within our body, such as metabolism, growth, development and reproduction. *Qi* is a moving force that is regulated and controlled by the Liver, so it plays a critical role in all aspects involving movement, such as the events surrounding ovulation and the motility of sperm. *Qi* (energy) is the expression of *jing* (essence) in *qi* form. Without it, conception and procreation are not possible.

THE FUNCTION OF *SHEN*

Shen is connected to the mind, consciousness and spirit, encompassing individual personality, feeling and thought. It is generated by the Heart and is nourished by Blood. It is reflected in the eyes, which are clear and vital when *shen* is healthy, dull and listless when *shen* is depleted.

Shen can be classified into two kinds: emotional and mental. Emotional *shen* refers to changes of mood, including joy, grief and anger, while mental *shen* refers to consciousness and thinking.

Mood changes are the responses of people to their surroundings. If unregulated, they will cause stagnation of *qi* and Blood, and disharmony between the internal organs, leading to illness and disease. It is therefore important to preserve a state of *shen* that is peaceful, tranquil and free from excessive desires and distracting thoughts.

Because *shen* controls thinking and memory, it also controls all the activities of the body. Since *shen* contributes to the smooth performance of all bodily functions that govern life and the physiological functions of the body as a whole, *shen* is also fundamentally important for fertility.

Shen is fully present in a baby before birth. Sound *shen* is considered to be the basis of health and longevity, so taking care of it is very important.

According to historical records, those who live a long life are almost always people who are adept at controlling their moods, by engaging in activities to ease the mind and finding a proper outlet for their emotions. This can include taking up hobbies such as playing the piano or chess, venting sorrow with a good cry, or confiding in others concerning the bitterness or grievance one feels. By releasing emotions, spirits are raised, intelligence is increased and circulation of *qi* and Blood are activated.

Thus the Three Treasures – *jing*, *qi* and *shen* – make up our constitution and represent an interaction between the body, mind and spirit. Although we cannot determine our basic constitution, we can positively affect our Three Treasures through the way we live our lives, thus maintaining balanced bodily functions and a harmonious mind.

The Five Elements (*Wu Xing*)

In Chinese philosophy, everything is related. The universe functions as an integrated whole, and we are a part of that whole. When one aspect (the *yin* or the *yang*) is out of balance, it has an impact on everything else. It is the nature of the universe to try to stay in balance at all times – so when there is an excess in one area, a corresponding deficiency will arise in another area.

Within the integrated whole, the world is composed of the Five Elements – wood, fire, earth, metal and water. Everything we know relates to one of these elements, including the different parts of the human body. Many people will be familiar with the importance of the elements in Feng Shui or astrology.

The interrelationships between the Five Elements are like those between the seasons of the year: balancing and checking one another, but also supporting and nourishing each other. Just as the rain of winter gives birth to the growth of spring, so the water of the elements promotes wood, wood promotes fire, and so on. Each of the elements has a generating or restraining effect on the next element in the cycle.

Generating

- Wood nourishes Fire
- Fire nourishes Earth
- Earth nourishes Metal
- Metal nourishes Water
- Water nourishes Wood

Restraining

- Wood overcomes Earth
- Earth overcomes Water
- Water overcomes Fire
- Fire overcomes Metal
- Metal overcomes Wood

The relationship between the Five Elements and the organs in the body.

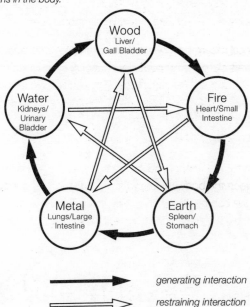

THE FIVE ELEMENTS AND THE BODY'S ORGANS

Like everything else in the world, each of the major organs of the body is classified according to which of the five elements it represents.

Wood – Liver/Gall Bladder

Fire – Heart/Small Intestine

Earth – Spleen/Stomach

Metal – Lungs/Large Intestine

Water – Kidneys/Urinary Bladder

Just as the diagram on page 25 symbolizes the relationship between the Five Elements, so it symbolizes the way the organs of the body relate to one another. The organs and tissues of the human body work in a similarly interdependent way as the Five Elements, nourishing or restraining each other's functions in the sequence and pattern shown in the diagram. TCM uses the interacting qualities of the elements to explain the physiology and causes of disease in the human body, and to guide diagnosis and treatment.

For example, wood generates fire. Fire is moderated by water, which comes from the Kidneys. So, if the Kidney *yin* (water) is insufficient to generate the Liver (wood), then Liver Heat will rise. That will, in turn, influence the Heart (fire) and Heat will rise there as well (causing insomnia). Another way it may be expressed is, the Liver is the *mother* of the Heart and the *child* of the Kidneys. In that way the influences are interrelated.

In relation to fertility, if Liver (wood) disharmony causes irregular periods, we need to consider whether this disharmony may be being affected by Heart (fire), that is, emotional causes, or whether it is due to the failure of Lungs (metal) to control Spleen (earth), which would then be unable to transform the fluids to support the Liver (wood) function.

However, it is not a rigid formula and in modern TCM, the Five Elements are just one of many ways of reading and understanding the workings of the human body.

The *zang* and *fu* organs of the body

When a TCM practitioner begins a diagnosis he or she will use 'organ phenomenon' theory to view the whole body, which encompasses the anatomy, physiology, pathology, type identification and healing principles of the main organs. Organ phenomenon theory is widely used in diagnosis and treatment and it associates the properties of the organs and tissues with the Five Elements (see above).

The five major solid organs of the body (Heart, Liver, Spleen, Lungs, Kidneys) are classified as *zang* (*yin*). The Pericardium can also be considered to be a *zang* organ. Each *zang* organ has a complementary *fu* (*yang*) organ and is associated with one of the five senses (Sight, Sound, Touch, Taste, Smell). All of this makes up a complex and integrated network in the body. This philosophy is central to the practice of acupuncture too, as explained further on page 38.

It is important to remember that the *zang* and *fu* organs are conceptual and bear little relation to their anatomical counterparts; they include spiritual and emotional components as well as physical.

THE *ZANG* ORGANS

The *zang* organs are considered to be *yin* and are divided into:

• Greater *yin* (*Taiyin*) – Lungs, Spleen
• Lesser *yin* (*Shaoyin*) – Heart, Kidneys
• Absolute *yin* (*Jueyin*) – Liver, Pericardium

Each of the *zang* organs has a specific function that relates to the other organs and tissues of the body. Using the diagnostic tools (see pages 31–33), your practitioner will identify how well each of your organs is performing. As always in TCM, the aim is to restore balance and harmony wherever they have been lost in the body.

The Heart

The Heart governs the Blood and vessels. The Heart circulates Blood constantly inside the vessels to supply nutrition to the whole body. If the Heart *qi* and Blood are sufficient, the heartbeat is regular, the pulse is harmonious and forceful, and the facial complexion is pink and lustrous. If the Heart *qi* and Blood are deficient, the Blood stagnates, which will present itself in a purple facial complexion, chills in the four limbs, restlessness, palpitations, insomnia and sleep that is disturbed by dreams. In pregnancy, this links to bleeding during pregnancy and therefore Blood deficiency.

The Lungs

Together with the Spleen, Kidneys, Intestines and Urinary Bladder, the Lungs are responsible for regulating the metabolism of water in the human body. The role of the Lungs in the metabolism of water can be described as clearing and regulating the waterways by conveying water downwards to the Urinary Bladder where it is excreted and distributing fluids throughout the body, particularly to the skin. If the Lungs fail to disperse fluids properly, a person may feel puffy or have difficulty urinating. This is due to Phlegm-Damp (see page 125). During pregnancy, this commonly shows in the form of swollen legs.

The Kidneys

The Kidneys are the foundation of the other organs; they store the 'essence' and govern growth, development and reproduction. The *qi* stored in the Kidneys is derived from the reproductive essence (*jing*, see page 23) inherited from the parents, which is the primitive substance needed for the development of the embryo.

From childhood, the essence in the Kidneys gradually develops and reaches its fullness in puberty when reproductive function reaches maturity and men are able to produce sperm and women are able to ovulate. The Kidneys play a major role in the urinary and reproductive systems, as well as in parts of the endocrine and nervous systems, more specifically in egg and sperm production.

If the essence-storing function of the Kidneys is impaired, growth, development and reproductive ability will be affected, possibly leading to infertility. The *yin* and *yang* of the Kidneys are mutually interdependent and keep the dynamic balance inside the human body. If this balance is disturbed, certain symptoms can develop such as night sweats, cold limbs, breathlessness, exhaustion, frequent urination, impotence and premature ejaculation in men, and infertility in women.

A pattern of early miscarriages usually has a genetic root and is linked to chromosomal make-up. In TCM, premature birth is thought to contribute to weakness in the Kidneys (which is related to our constitution at birth).

The Liver
The Liver governs the free, uninterrupted flow of vital energy within the human body. In TCM, this key organ is considered to have the same functions and roles as those in Western medicine. The Liver also maintains and stores blood, which is regarded as 'reproductive essence'. It regulates the amount of blood which the various parts of the body need, and therefore has a great influence over menstrual cycles in women, as well as the Kidney's essence (see above).

The Liver is also responsible for promoting a well-balanced circulation of the *qi* energy in the body. This influences the metabolism or dispersion of body fluids. It is this harmonious balance between the Liver and the Kidneys that is believed to play a very important part in assisting successful ovulation and consequent conception.

Generally speaking, the Liver *yin* should control the Liver *yang* to prevent it from being hyperactive. If the Liver *yin* becomes insufficient and fails to restrain the Liver *yang*, the Liver *yang*'s hyperactivity then most commonly causes premenstrual tension, short temper and headaches. On the other hand, when the Liver *qi* is suppressed, symptoms such as depression, sadness, sore breasts and diarrhoea will develop.

In relation to pregnancy, if the Liver *yang* is overactive it may cause severe morning sickness, or high blood pressure during the later stages of pregnancy.

The Spleen
Blood and postnatal *qi* energy originate from the Spleen, and are the foundation for life after birth. The Spleen governs transportation and transformation and provides the necessary nourishment for healthy growth that transform *qi* and Blood. The functions of the Spleen include digestion, absorption and distribution. Therefore, when there

are problems with the Spleen, there will be an accumulation of Damp and Phlegm due to fluid retention. This can sometimes lead to obstructions within the abdomen and problems such as abdominal distension, diarrhoea and nutritional disturbance. It can also result in poor blood flow in the reproductive system, tubal obstructions and endometriosis. Consequently, the healthy development of the egg or sperm will be hindered. In pregnancy, problems with the Spleen may lead to malnourishment of the foetus during development.

The Pericardium

The Pericardium displays many of the same functions as the Heart. In TCM it is usually only referred to in the case of infectious diseases caused by external Heat.

THE *FU* ORGANS

The *fu* organs are *yang* and are divided into:

- Greater *yang* (*Taiyang*) – Small Intestine, Urinary Bladder
- Lesser *yang* (*Shaoyang*) – Triple Burner, Gall Bladder
- *Yang* Brightness (*Yangming*) – Large Intestine, Stomach

The Fu organs are considered to be hollow vessels which can receive or expel the nutrients, energy or waste generated by the *zang* organs. Each of the *fu* organs is paired with a corresponding *zang* organ.

The Small Intestine

The Small Intestine is paired with the Heart. It receives and stores water and food.

The Urinary Bladder

The Urinary Bladder is paired with the Kidneys and stores and excretes urine. Problems with Kidney *qi* will show up in urinary problems.

The Triple Burner

The Triple Burner (*San Jiao*) is paired with the Pericardium, which encases the Heart.

- *The Upper Burner*, located above the diaphragm, assists the functions of the Heart and Lungs.
- *The Middle Burner*, located between the diaphragm and the navel, assists the functions of the Stomach and Spleen.
- *The Lower Burner*, located below the navel, assists the functions of the Kidneys and Urinary Bladder.

The Gall Bladder

The Gall Bladder stores and excretes bile. It is paired with the Liver. Together they control the Blood and our *qi* levels.

The Large Intestine

The Large Intestine is paired with the Lungs and deals with the body's solid waste. The Large Intestine's ability to absorb water affects whether we suffer loose bowels (too little absorption) or constipation (too much absorption.)

The Stomach

The Stomach is paired with the Spleen. If Stomach *qi* is weak, food stagnates and digestive problems will develop.

The constitution

According to traditional Chinese practice, there are both internal and external causes of health problems and disease (see pages 102–103). Broadly speaking, any kind of extreme stimulation or emotional suppression will interrupt *qi* (energy flow) and will have a resulting impact on the essential organs of the body.

The external causes are known as the Six Excesses: Wind, Cold, Heat, Damp, Dryness and Fire.

The internal causes are known as the Seven Emotions: Joy, Anger, Anxiety, Pensiveness, Sorrow, Fear, Fright.

This is the language of diagnosis in TCM. For example, the pages that follow explain, especially, the need to reduce Heat in the body. I will use words like Moist, Cold, Dry and so on to describe physical symptoms. The language may seem a little strange at first but you will find you soon develop an instinctive understanding of the terminology because it relates to the natural world and therefore 'makes sense'.

THE SIX EXCESSES

As we have seen, there are six climatic states in the natural world – Wind, Cold, Heat, Damp, Dryness and Fire. These are also known as *environmental qi*. Under normal circumstances, they do not cause disease. Only when the climate changes abruptly or when the body's resistance is low, may these become excesses that disrupt the human body and cause problems or disease.

Wind	Attacks through the body	Injures Blood and *yin*
Cold	Attacks from the skin	Injures Kidney *yang*
Heat	Clouds the mind and skin	Injures the *yin*
Damp	Impairs digestion	Injures Spleen *yang*

| **Dryness** | Impairs the balance of fluids | Injures Blood and *yin* |
| **Fire** | Forces the body to change | Depletes Blood and *yin* |

THE SEVEN EMOTIONS

In TCM it is understood that extreme emotional changes can have an impact on the internal organs. Seven core emotions have been identified that describe basic human mental and emotional states. They are: feeling overjoyed, extreme anger, Anxiety, Pensiveness, Sorrow, Fear, Fright.

Under normal circumstances, emotions ebb and flow; they are transitory and unlikely to cause any problems. However, if a persistent emotional state or sudden and intense mental trauma occurs, it may cause dysfunction within the body and have an impact on the *yin*, *yang*, *qi*, Blood and internal organs, which will in turn lead to disease.

Some common symptoms caused by the emotions are: insomnia or disturbed sleep, palpitations, depression, irritable bowel syndrome, a sensation of obstruction in the throat and menstrual irregularities.

Joy	Damages the Heart	Reduces *qi*
Anger	Injures the Liver	Stimulates *qi*
Anxiety	Harms the Lungs	Obstructs *qi*
Pensiveness	Affects the Spleen	Blocks *qi*
Sorrow	Affects the Lungs	Reduces *qi*
Fear	Injures the Kidneys	Suppresses *qi*
Fright	Affects the Heart and may also affect the Kidneys	Disrupts *qi*

TCM diagnostic techniques

TCM practitioners view the human body differently from their Western medical colleagues so the diagnosis of infertility will use different diagnostic tools and will look for specific physical manifestations.

There are four key diagnostic tools in TCM:

- Questioning
- Observing
- Listening (to the body)
- Smelling

These are used with the more precise tools of tongue diagnosis and reading the pulse.

When you meet a TCM practitioner he or she will ask you questions and examine you. Their diagnosis and treatment strategy will depend on their assessment of the involvement and balance of relationships between the internal organs. They will also take into consideration your constitution (habits), external environment, appearance of the tongue, pulse, diet, mind and lifestyle before reaching a conclusion.

Just as TCM uses different treatment methods from Western medicine, including herbs and acupuncture, so it uses different diagnostic techniques. It looks at the body as a whole, examining the different physical signs and symptoms before treatment. Treatment is tailored to each patient individually as every case is different.

DIAGNOSING FERTILITY PROBLEMS

When you visit a TCM practitioner to discuss your fertility problems you will be asked for a full history of your menstrual cycle, diet, bowel habits, a general health profile and any tests you may already have undertaken with your doctor. It is important that both you and your partner attend the initial consultation as the TCM practitioner has to identify whether there is a need to treat only the woman or whether to treat both of you.

A TCM practitioner will also perform specific examinations that you may not have experienced before. These are non-invasive processes and will help the practitioner build a profile of *your pattern type* (see page 117–135); any *excesses* and *deficiencies* (see pages 104–112) in your body and how to target the treatment plan to rebalance the causes of your fertility problems.

Physical inspection

The practitioner will observe your general and local physical condition, including your facial complexion, your body, the motion and coating of your tongue and your spirit and general bearing.

Tongue diagnosis

In TCM the tongue is regarded as a strong indicator of imbalance or illness and a qualified practitioner will look at your tongue for signs of syndromes that may be affecting your fertility. Each portion of the tongue – tip, sides, middle and back – corresponds to different internal organs, as the diagram opposite shows.

Colour is an important sign as tongues can vary from very pale to deep purplish, depending on whether you have an excess of Heat or Cold.

- Purplish and moist   Extreme Cold, Blood stagnation
- Dark red   Extreme Heat syndrome, *yin* deficiency
- Purplish and dry   Extreme Heat, *yin* and fluid deficiency
- Pale   Cold syndrome, *yang* deficiency, *qi* deficiency, Blood deficiency

Each portion of the tongue – tip, sides, middle and back – corresponds to different internal organs.

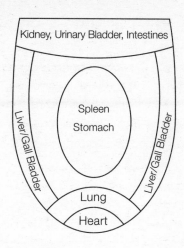

Kidney, Urinary Bladder, Intestines

Spleen
Stomach

Liver/Gall Bladder

Liver/Gall Bladder

Lung

Heart

The coating on the surface of the tongue is another reflection of internal health: it should be thin, moist and white. If the coating looks thick and white, or yellowish, it suggests there is a problem with the organ associated with that specific area of the tongue.

- Yellow coating   Heat syndrome
- White coating   Cold syndrome

It is the combination of these physical aspects that will help a practitioner diagnose your condition and it requires a great deal of skill and experience to read the signs.

Reading the pulse

Pulse diagnosis is vital. The meridians of the human body act as pathways for the circulation of *qi* and Blood, and as *qi* and Blood are dominated by the Heart it is therefore possible to understand the state of *qi* and Blood and the constitution of the human body by feeling for pulses. Although Western doctors will feel your pulse at the wrist they are looking simply to count and measure your heart rate. TCM doctors use the pace, texture and strength of pulses to detect internal problems.

A TCM doctor will press, using three fingers, to measure different pulse spots on both of your wrists, at a variety of surface depths. The pulse response is classified under specific terms such as *normal, floating, deep, slow, rapid, slippery, choppy, wiry, weak, floating, solid* or *full*. These terms are used very precisely in TCM and determine a much broader range of symptoms and conditions than the Western method.

The TCM doctor will assess the pulse diagnosis in combination with the results of the other diagnostic methods to see what type emerges (see pages 117–135). All the organs of the body are taken into account to develop a full picture of a patient's overall fertility. Please see pages 251–258 for the detailed diagnostic questionnaire that I give to all my patients.

TCM TREATMENT IS NOT A GUARANTEE OF SUCCESS

Unfortunately, not everyone who longs for a baby is able to become pregnant. For those who find it is not to be, the realization can be acutely painful and distressing. This is why we go to some lengths to ensure that there are no functional problems underlying the fertility problem before we begin treatment. It is important that we don't raise people's hopes if the odds are not in their favour.

My heart goes out to those patients whose results are consistently negative. So many of the couples we see are committed to their treatment programme and do everything we advise. More often than not, when a baby does not result, it is because time is no longer on the woman's side; it is rarely to do with something the couple have or haven't done – though people too often blame themselves. We try to offer support and can provide herbal remedies to help ease personal distress and help to rebalance the body – but sadly, the sense of loss and grief take longer to heal.

Chapter 2

THE PRINCIPLES OF ACUPUNCTURE

Most people in the West are familiar with acupuncture these days. In fact, many people who visit a physiotherapist or even their family doctor may be offered a form of acupuncture to help with aches and pains in their knees, back or neck. Although some areas of the Western medical establishment are still cautious about recommending it, acupuncture is widely respected – especially in the treatment of unexplained and persistent lower back pain.

Acupuncture is a complex and highly specialized treatment method that goes right to the heart of the body's internal and external networks. And because it treats the ways different parts of the body relate to one another, it is very effective in treating fertility problems by tackling the interrelationships of hormones, Blood and *qi* before and during a pregnancy. It is even more effective when used alongside Chinese herbal medicine.

Scientific trials on acupuncture

A lot of attention has been focused in recent years on the use of acupuncture in IVF treatments, in particular on the practice of treating women with acupuncture on the day of their egg collection and on the day the fertilized eggs are transferred. Several trials have been completed but they have shown conflicting and confusing results. Many show an improvement in the successful pregnancy and live birth rate if acupuncture is used, others find no such improvement.

One particular report received a lot of publicity when it was published in March 2010. The British Fertility Society published an overview of trials that had been done on the use of acupuncture, given on the day of egg collection, on the day of implantation, and again a few days later. The report stated: No matter at which point in the process acupuncture was given, there was no significant difference in the live birth rate, clinical pregnancy rate or miscarriage rate between patients that had received acupuncture and those that had not.

'The British Fertility Society concludes that there is currently no evidence that acupuncture or Chinese herbal medicine when used in conjunction with assisted fertility treatment, have any beneficial effect on live birth rate, pregnancy rate or miscarriage rate.' (*British Fertility Society issues new guidelines on the use of acupuncture and herbal medicine in fertility treatment*, British Fertility Society Press Release, 10 March 2010.)

For any experienced practitioner of TCM this conclusion made no sense. Medical 'double-blind' trials are based on the clinical results of two groups of patients. In one group, every patient receives exactly the same treatment and number of doses. The second group receives identical placebo (non-medical) treatment. No one involved knows which patients are receiving the medical treatment and which are receiving the placebo. The results of the two groups are then compared, to assess and measure the efficacy of the medical treatment.

But it is not appropriate to use this kind of trial to assess the effect of TCM because a TCM doctor will diagnose and treat each patient as an individual, even if two patients are diagnosed with the same condition. That is, the external symptoms may be the same, but the underlying cause is likely to be different, which means the treatment will vary from patient to patient. Likewise, there is no correlation between the *number* of acupuncture sessions and an increased chance of successful fertility treatment. Each treatment is administered for a particular reason. So an acupuncture trial in which all the patients receive the same treatment makes no sense to a TCM doctor. (I have also since wondered whether the trial may have mistakenly considered acupuncture on its own to be synonymous with Chinese Herbal Medicine as a medical discipline, as the trial did not involve treating patients with Chinese herbs at all.)

A successful fertility treatment that incorporates the use of acupuncture with or without Chinese herbs is a treatment that needs to be given for some weeks or months in advance of IVF. It is a preparation for pregnancy that improves egg quality and the woman's abdominal environment for successful implantation. It is not something that can affect the outcome on one day.

Of course, acupuncture *can* play a specific role on the day. Egg collection punctures the ovary and can cause inflammation of the abdomen; acupuncture can treat the increased blood flow. And it can also help relax the woman in advance of implantation, which is also important. But this, in my estimate, could only improve the success rate by 3 to 4 per cent. This is based on the assumption that the egg and sperm are of good quality and the woman has a healthy abdominal blood flow.

I feel very strongly that this is one of the areas in which Western medicine uses inappropriate testing methods. Acupuncture is not a quick fix on the day. It should be carefully tailored to improve a patient's fertility potential before IVF treatment is given. And, like many experts in the field, I know that TCM works not only for women. Acupuncture and herbal medicine also have an impressive success rate in improving male sperm count, motility and quality.

So, having stated my position, and that of most leading acupuncture specialists, let's look at what acupuncture is and what it can do.

What is acupuncture?

Put simply, acupuncture is the insertion of hair-fine needles into the body at a great variety of different points and to a variety of different depths, depending on the problems diagnosed. The places where the needles are inserted, the acupuncture points, are linked by underlying networks with a complex and sophisticated theory behind them.

This system of therapy has been in constant use throughout China for over 2,500 years, with its history dating back to the middle of the Chou Period (6th century BC). Before the introduction of metal needles, practitioners probably used thorns, sharp splinters of bamboo or picks made of animal horn, before moving on to sharpened stones and bones. Iron needles were first brought into use in the Han Period (about 160 BC).

As with herbal treatments, the system that underpins acupuncture was first documented in the *Huang Di Nei Jing*, the Yellow Emperor's classic volume of internal medicine (see page 14), the oldest and most famous of the Chinese medical classics. The idea of a system of meridians through which the *qi* circulates was well established by the time of the book's publication in 2700 BC, although the precise locations of acupuncture points on the body did not become standard until later.

It is interesting that the system of acupuncture we use today is actually a mixture of different methods from different areas of the Chinese Empire, each partly influenced by the different geography of the region in which it originated. So although acupuncture originated in the east, the use of nine needles of different shapes arose in the south. Chinese herbalism came more from the west, whereas moxibustion, which involves the burning of moxa (the herb mugwort) just above an acupuncture point to provide a heat stimulus, developed mainly in the cold north of China. The various treatments also had slightly different applications: acupuncture was thought generally more suitable for acute conditions, while moxa and Chinese herbs were considered a more effective treatment for chronic illness.

Acupuncture continued to develop and its systems became formalized and written down over the centuries. There is written evidence in text and on bronze statues that the full set of 365 acupuncture points (see page 53), which form the basis of modern acupuncture, were in use in the 15th century.

Since that time acupuncture has been studied and practised by masters of the discipline over many years, so the system in use today is a highly evolved and well-developed doctrine.

The basic principles

Acupuncture is concerned mainly with improving the flow of *qi* through the body, stimulating, balancing and moving it. It can help restore balance between the *zang* and *fu* organs (see pages 26–30).

The body contains a number of main meridians or channels (*jing*) and branches (*luo*), which form a network of pathways that transport *qi* and Blood, and connect the internal organs with other parts of the body and with the outside of the body. The actual acupuncture points along these meridians, which we'll look at later, represent openings in the meridians through which the flow of *qi* can be altered.

The network of pathways is like the nervous system or the blood circulatory system in the body, except that the meridians cannot be seen, they connect through energy alone.

No one knows precisely how acupuncture works, although there are many interpretations. The Western interpretation is that the meridians are electrical pathways running through the body and that the stimulation by needles at certain points amplifies the current. Other researchers believe that the needles stimulate the body's nervous system to release chemicals, which relieve pain and carry messages back to the brain so that it releases 'feel-good' endorphins.

Acupuncture is used in fertility treatment on women to stimulate reactions in the body that support the function of the pituitary gland, which controls the ovaries, adrenal and thyroid glands. This stimulates the body to balance its secretion of hormones. In male fertility treatment, acupuncture has proved to be a highly successful method of raising sperm count, motility and quality.

Although acupuncture is a complex system, it is interesting to understand how your body works as an integrated whole and to learn how you can use acupressure yourself to help support your treatment (see pages 225–232).

THE MAIN MERIDIANS

Although there are many meridians in the body, most treatments use the 12 main meridians that form the dominant or Primary system. They are arranged in six pairs of complementary *yin* and *yang* meridians. They connect the internal organs to the external parts of the body, allowing the human body to function as an organic whole. This is why you can stimulate a point in the arm or feet to affect the working of the Kidney or ovaries, for example. The 12 meridians run vertically up and down the body, a full set on both sides of the centre line.

TCM recognizes the *yin* and *yang* within the internal organs in the body as outlined earlier on pages 26–30. Each *yin* organ is associated with a *yang* organ and one of the five elements, and these associations are reflected in the Primary Meridians.

The *yin* organs	The *yang* organs
Lungs (metal)	Large Intestine (metal)
Spleen (earth)	Stomach (earth)
Heart (fire)	Small Intestine (fire)
Kidneys (water)	Urinary Bladder (water)
Liver (wood)	Gall Bladder (wood)
Pericardium (fire)	Triple Burner (fire)

The Primary Meridians

There are 12 main meridians, each replicated on both sides of the body. They are divided into six pairs, each with a *yang* and *yin* meridian. *Yang* meridians or channels are on the external sides of the limbs while *yin* meridians are on the internal sides. Quite often, the meridians relating to the *yang* organ will be used to treat disorders of its related *yin* organ.

Not all acupuncture points are used for fertility treatment. The points marked on the diagrams in this section are those I have found to be useful for acupuncture and/or acupressure. They are referred to and explained in the treatment chapters. (The points marked in grey are the start and end points for each meridian and are provided for reference.) A qualified TCM practitioner may choose to use other points relevant to the needs of the individual patient. The following diagrams are representative of the meridians as a whole and do not show the detail in all instances.

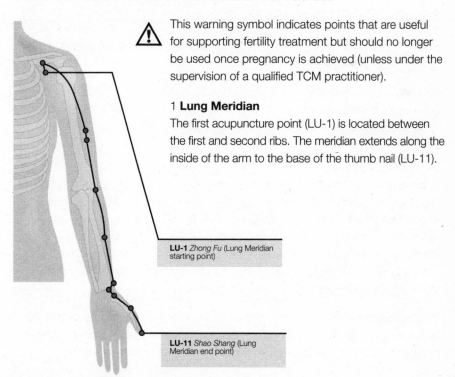

This warning symbol indicates points that are useful for supporting fertility treatment but should no longer be used once pregnancy is achieved (unless under the supervision of a qualified TCM practitioner).

1 Lung Meridian

The first acupuncture point (LU-1) is located between the first and second ribs. The meridian extends along the inside of the arm to the base of the thumb nail (LU-11).

LU-1 *Zhong Fu* (Lung Meridian starting point)

LU-11 *Shao Shang* (Lung Meridian end point)

2 Large Intestine Meridian

This begins at the base of the nail of the index finger (LI-1). It extends along the upper side of the arm to the shoulder and ends at a midpoint on the outer curve of the nostril (LI-20), where it links up with the Stomach Meridian.

The Lungs (*yin*) are paired with the Large Intestine (*yang*). Their entry point is the nose, and they govern the skin and hair.

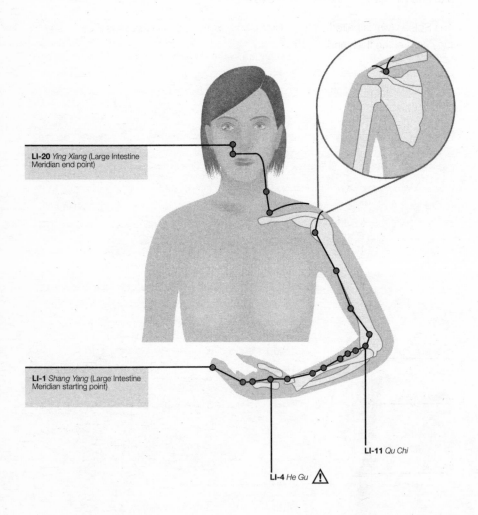

LI-20 *Ying Xiang* (Large Intestine Meridian end point)

LI-1 *Shang Yang* (Large Intestine Meridian starting point)

LI-11 *Qu Chi*

LI-4 *He Gu*

3 Stomach Meridian

Beginning at the lateral side of the nose, the Stomach Meridian ascends to the medial side of the eye and then descends to below the pupil beneath the eye to emerge at ST-1. It then follows along the nose before entering the upper gums. It curves around the lips and runs along the lower jaw before ascending in front of the ear to the forehead. A branch separates at ST-5 and descends down along the throat region towards the clavicle at ST-12 and crosses to the upper back. At ST-12 a further branch descends to the breast and abdomen. It extends downwards through the leg and ends at the tip of the second toe (ST-45).

The Spleen (*yin*) is paired with the Stomach (*yang*). Their entry point is the mouth and they control the flesh and the limbs.

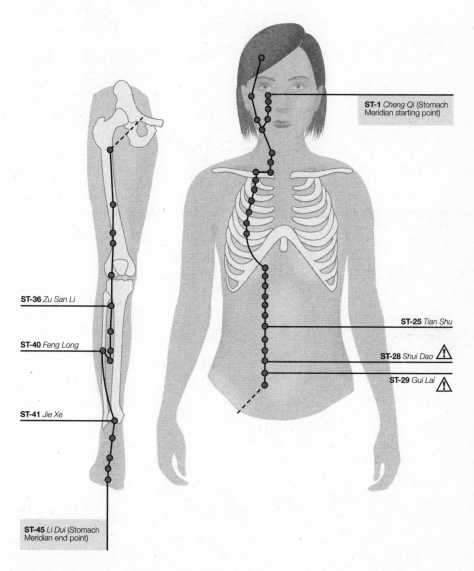

ST-1 *Cheng Qi* (Stomach Meridian starting point)

ST-36 *Zu San Li*

ST-40 *Feng Long*

ST-41 *Jie Xe*

ST-45 *Li Dui* (Stomach Meridian end point)

ST-25 *Tian Shu*

ST-28 *Shui Dao* ⚠

ST-29 *Gui Lai* ⚠

4 Spleen Meridian

This begins at the tip of the big toe (SP-1). From there it travels along the outside edge of the foot and up the leg, past the knee and the thigh to the abdomen, where it enters the spleen and stomach. From there it ascends to the Lung Meridian starting point (LU-1), located between the first and second ribs, then descends to terminate at *Da Bao* (SP-21), located in the seventh intercostal space on the mid-axillary line. A branch ascends alongside the oesophagus and spreads over the lower surface of the tongue.

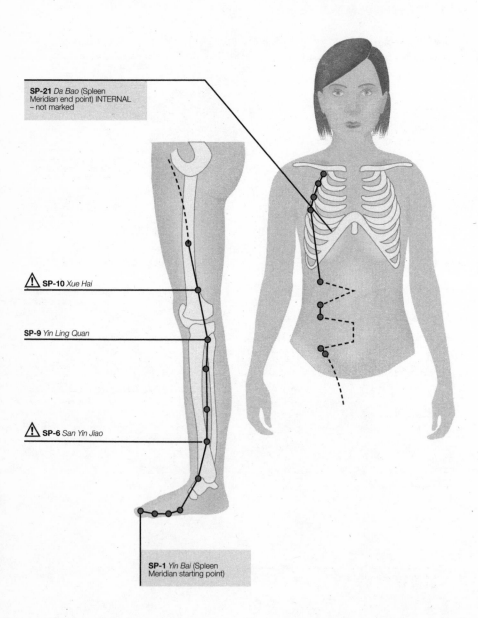

SP-21 *Da Bao* (Spleen Meridian end point) INTERNAL – not marked

SP-10 *Xue Hai*

SP-9 *Yin Ling Quan*

SP-6 *San Yin Jiao*

SP-1 *Yin Bai* (Spleen Meridian starting point)

5 Heart Meridian

The Heart meridian originates in the Heart and connects to the Small Intestine. It emerges in the centre of the armpit at acupuncture point H-1 and continues along the inner arm to the wrist and ends at the tip of the little finger (H-9).

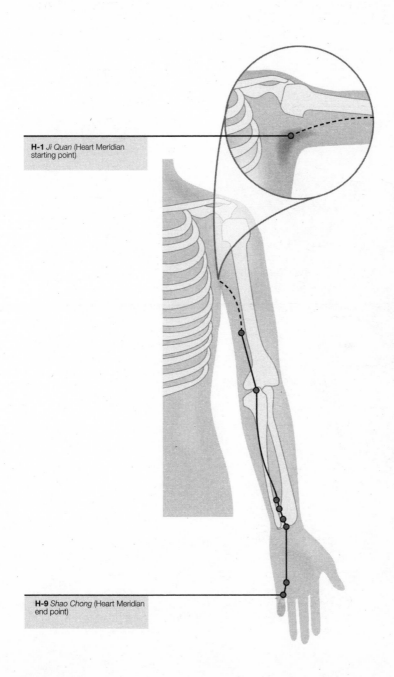

H-1 *Ji Quan* (Heart Meridian starting point)

H-9 *Shao Chong* (Heart Meridian end point)

6 Small Intestine Meridian

This begins on the outside edge of the little finger (SI-1) and continues up the edge of the hand to the curve by the wrist bone. It ascends along the outside of the arm to the outer shoulder blade. It then zigzags across the shoulder blade to the face, ending by the ear (SI-19).

The Heart (*yin*) is paired with the Small Intestine (*yang*). Their entry point is the tongue. They control the blood vessels and show in the face.

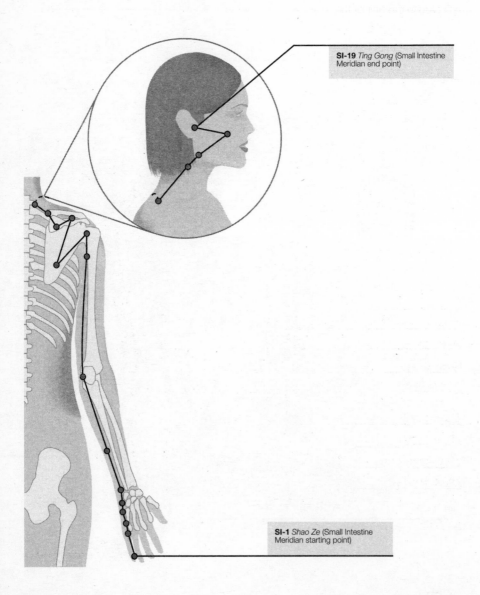

SI-19 *Ting Gong* (Small Intestine Meridian end point)

SI-1 *Shao Ze* (Small Intestine Meridian starting point)

7 **Urinary Bladder Meridian**

This begins in the inside corner of the eye (UB-1) and ascends to the forehead and the temple, where it enters the brain, reappearing at the nape of the neck. It then continues down the back, following a line adjacent to the spine, across the buttock to the side of the thigh and down the back of the thigh to the back of the knee. It then travels back up to the shoulder blade, following a slightly different route. The meridian then runs down the back again, where it meets itself at the knee, then continues down the leg to the outer tip of the little toe (UB-67) (see page 234).

The Kidneys (*yin*) are paired with the Urinary Bladder (*yang*). Their entry points are the ear and the urethra. They control the brain, bones and marrow, and their health is reflected in the hair of the head.

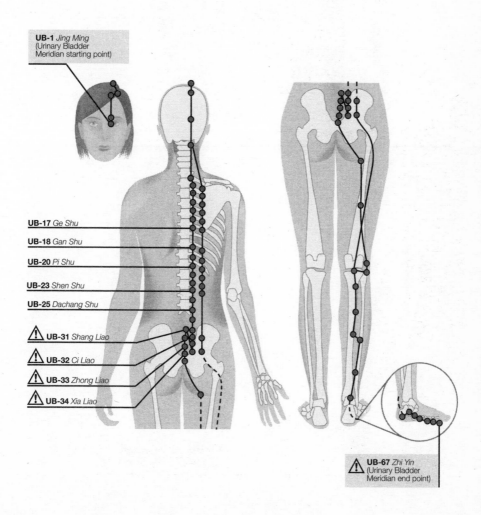

UB-1 *Jing Ming*
(Urinary Bladder
Meridian starting point)

UB-17 *Ge Shu*

UB-18 *Gan Shu*

UB-20 *Pi Shu*

UB-23 *Shen Shu*

UB-25 *Dachang Shu*

⚠ **UB-31** *Shang Liao*

⚠ **UB-32** *Ci Liao*

⚠ **UB-33** *Zhong Liao*

⚠ **UB-34** *Xia Liao*

⚠ **UB-67** *Zhi Yin*
(Urinary Bladder
Meridian end point)

8 Kidney Meridian

The Kidney Meridian begins beneath the little toe and runs along the sole of the foot. The first acupuncture point is KID-1, between the second and third toes in the depression below the ball of the foot. It runs up the inside of the leg via the inner thigh to the pubic bone. It ascends along the lumbar spine. The final acupuncture point is KID-27 on the lower border of the clavicle.

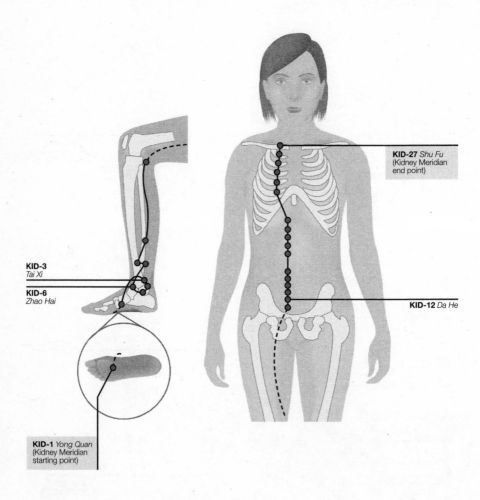

KID-27 *Shu Fu*
(Kidney Meridian
end point)

KID-3
Tai Xi

KID-6
Zhao Hai

KID-12 *Da He*

KID-1 *Yong Quan*
(Kidney Meridian
starting point)

9 Pericardium Meridian

The Pericardium Meridian originates in the chest. The first acupuncture point is just on the outside of the nipple (PC-1). It then moves towards the arm and down the inner arm to the wrist, ending at PC-9, the centre of the tip of the middle finger.

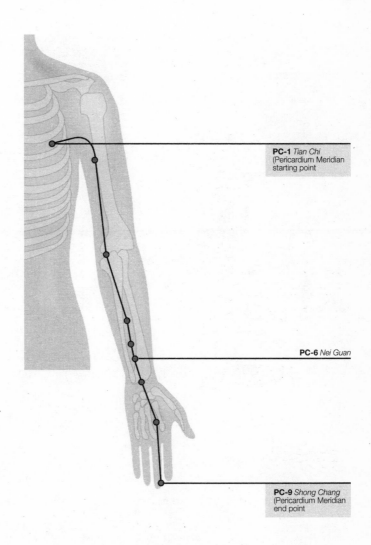

PC-1 *Tian Chi* (Pericardium Meridian starting point

PC-6 *Nei Guan*

PC-9 *Shong Chang* (Pericardium Meridian end point

10 Triple Burner Meridian

This begins on the outside edge of the fourth finger (TB-1 or SJ-1) and flows to the back of the wrist and up the back of the arm to the shoulder joint. A branch ascends along the neck to behind the ear and then circles the ear. Another branch separates behind the ear, crosses the face and ends at the eyebrow (TB-23 or SJ-23) where it links with the Gall Bladder Meridian.

The Pericardium (*yin*) is paired with the Triple Burner (*yang*).

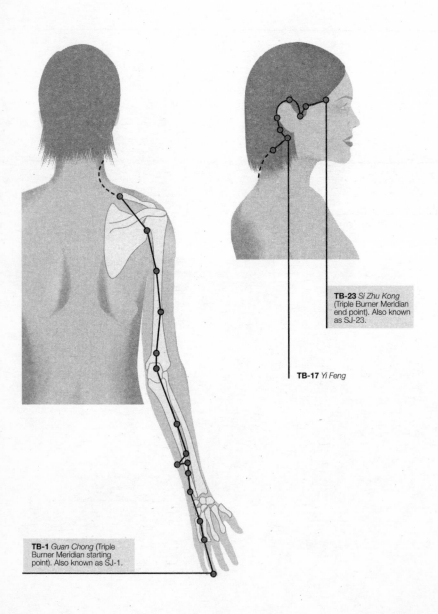

TB-23 *Si Zhu Kong* (Triple Burner Meridian end point). Also known as SJ-23.

TB-17 *Yi Feng*

TB-1 *Guan Chong* (Triple Burner Meridian starting point). Also known as SJ-1.

11 Gall Bladder Meridian

This begins at the outer hollow of the eye socket (GB-1), it curves around the ear to the forehead and then back down the skull to the shoulder. The meridian then descends through the chest to the lower ribs and downwards to the hip. It then descends along the outside leg and the edge of the foot, ending at the edge of the fourth toe (GB-44).

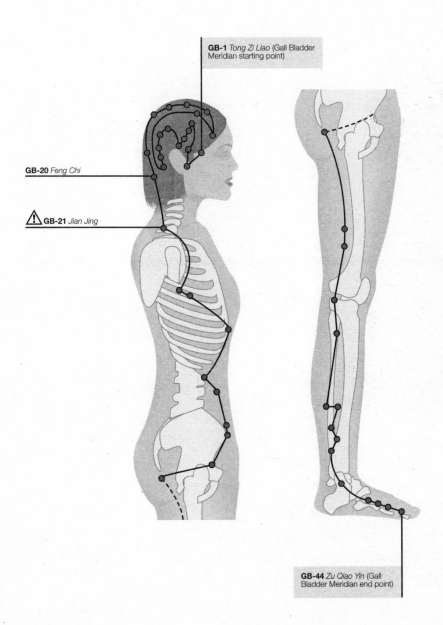

GB-1 *Tong Zi Liao* (Gall Bladder Meridian starting point)

GB-20 *Feng Chi*

⚠ **GB-21** *Jian Jing*

GB-44 *Zu Qiao Yin* (Gall Bladder Meridian end point)

12 Liver Meridian

The Liver Meridian begins at the big toe (LV-1) and runs across the top of the foot, up the calf via the inner thigh to the genital area. It continues upwards to the lower ribs, ending at a point below the nipple (LV-14).

The Liver (*yin*) is paired with the Gall Bladder (*yang*). Their entry point is the eyes. They control the sinews (muscles and joints), and their state of health shows in the nails of the fingers and toes.

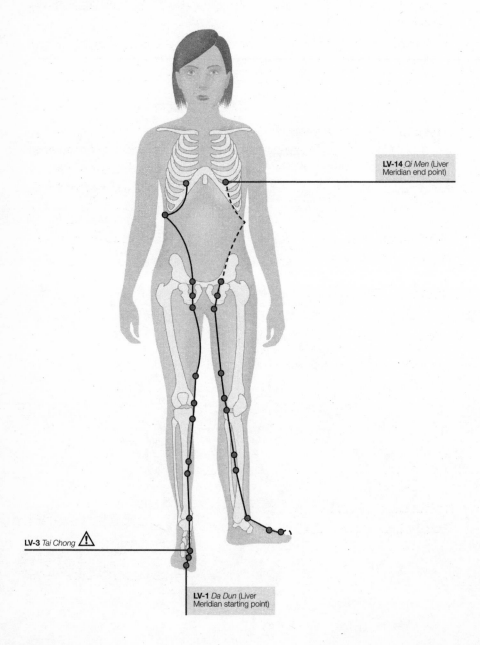

LV-14 *Qi Men* (Liver Meridian end point)

LV-3 *Tai Chong* ⚠️

LV-1 *Da Dun* (Liver Meridian starting point)

THE SMALLER MERIDIANS

The other meridians are branches of the main system, like tributaries flowing into main rivers. They include the Extraordinary Vessels, the Divergent Channels, the Collaterals, the Sinew Channels and the Skin.

Their four main functions are:

- To interconnect the internal organs and all tissues in the body.
- To allow *qi* and Blood to circulate throughout the whole body in an orderly flow to nourish the body and maintain the balance of *yin* and *yang*.
- To protect the body from attack by external disease and to signal symptoms and signs of internal imbalance or illness.
- To transmit the 'needling sensation' to diseased areas in order to regulate deficiency and excess that might be causing a problem.

The Extraordinary Vessels

Of the eight Extraordinary Vessels, three are particularly important in fertility treatment – the Conception Vessel, the Governing Vessel and the Penetrating Vessel. The Conception Vessel and the Governing Vessel are the only Extraordinary Vessels that have acupuncture points of their own.

The Conception Vessel (*Ren mai*) is *yin* in nature and runs straight up and down the midline of the body at the front.

The Conception Vessel

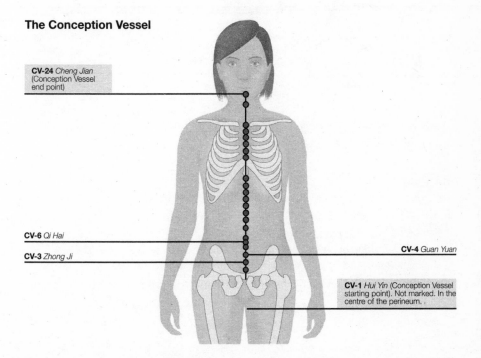

CV-24 *Cheng Jian* (Conception Vessel end point)

CV-6 *Qi Hai*

CV-3 *Zhong Ji*

CV-4 *Guan Yuan*

CV-1 *Hui Yin* (Conception Vessel starting point). Not marked. In the centre of the perineum.

The Governing Vessel (*Du mai*) is *yang* in nature and runs primarily up the spine at the back of the body.

The Governing Vessel

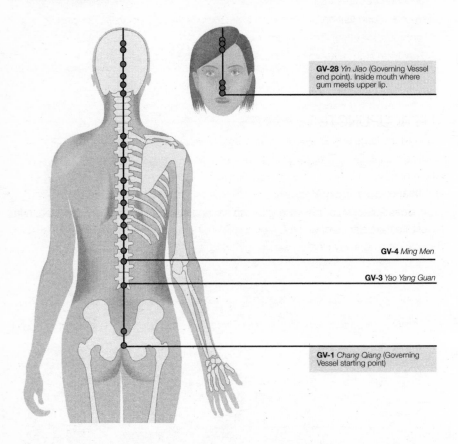

GV-28 *Yin Jiao* (Governing Vessel end point). Inside mouth where gum meets upper lip.

GV-4 *Ming Men*

GV-3 *Yao Yang Guan*

GV-1 *Chang Qiang* (Governing Vessel starting point)

The Conception Vessel and the Governing Vessel can be regarded as forming the polar axes of *yin* and *yang* of the body.

The Penetrating Vessel

The Penetrating Vessel (*Chong mai*) is an Extraordinary Vessel that has a particularly important role in fertility treatment. It influences the supply and movement of Blood in the uterus and has a deep influence on menstruation. This vessel originates in the pelvic cavity and ascends the front of the body as well as the spine. It has no acupuncture points of its own, but links the Stomach and Kidney Meridians, and helps to strengthen the connection between the Conception and Governing Vessels.

THE ACUPUNCTURE POINTS

Along all the large and small meridians there are specific acupuncture points where needles are inserted. These are the sites where *qi* and Blood are transported and where illness can invade the body. By stimulating these points it is possible to prevent and treat disease. The general principle of acupuncture and moxibustion treatment (see pages 233–234) at these specific sites is to regulate the flow of *qi* and Blood, and to restore the balance of *yin* and *yang* through either correcting deficiency, reducing excess, clearing away Heat or warming Cold.

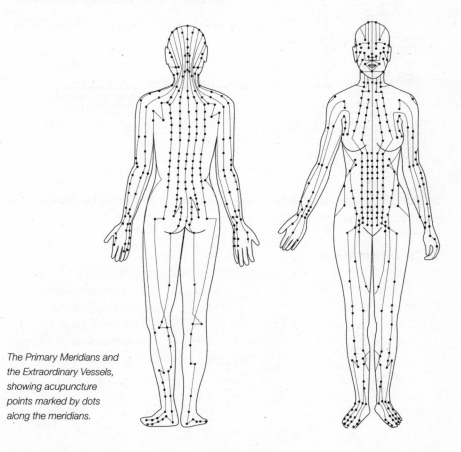

The Primary Meridians and the Extraordinary Vessels, showing acupuncture points marked by dots along the meridians.

ACUPUNCTURE CHART

⚠ Although useful for fertility treatment, these points should only be used during pregnancy under the supervision of a qualified TCM practitioner.

POINT	ABBREVIATION	WESTERN NAME	WARNING	NOTES
Conception vessel (*Ren mai*)				
Zhong Ji	CV-3	Middle Pole		
Guan Yuan	CV-4	Gateway to Original *Qi*		
Qi Hai	CV-6	Sea of *Qi*		
Governing vessel (*Du mai*)				
Yao Yang Guan	GV-3	Barrier of the *Yang*		Used for acupressure (pages 230–231)
Large Intestine Meridian				
He Gu	LI-4	Joining Valley	⚠	
Qu Chi	LI-11	Pool at the Bend		
Stomach Meridian				
Tian Shu	ST-25	Heaven's Pivot		Used for acupressure (pages 230–231)
Shui Dao	ST-28	Waterway	⚠	Used for acupressure (pages 230–231)
Gui Lai	ST-29	Return	⚠	Used for acupressure (pages 230–231)
Zu San Li	ST-36	Leg Three Miles		
Feng Long	ST-40	Abundant Bulge		
Jie Xi	ST-41	Stream Divide		
Spleen Meridian				
San Yin Jiao	SP-6	Three *Yin* Intersection	⚠	
Yin Ling Quan	SP-9	*Yin* Mound Spring		
Xue Hai	SP-10	Sea of Blood	⚠	
Urinary Bladder Meridian				
Ge Shu	UB-17	Diaphragm *Shu*		
Gan Shu	UB-18	Liver *Shu*		
Pi Shu	UB-20	Spleen *Shu*		
Shen Shu	UB-23	Kidney *Shu*		
Dachang Shu	UB-25	Large Intestine *Shu*		
Shang Liao	UB-31	Upper Crevice	⚠	Used for acupressure (pages 230–231)
Ci Liao	UB-32	Second Crevice	⚠	Used for acupressure (pages 230–231)
Zhong Liao	UB-33	Middle Crevice	⚠	Used for acupressure (pages 230–231)
Xia Liao	UB-34	Lower Crevice	⚠	Used for acupressure (pages 230–231)
Zhi Yin	UB-67	Reaching *Yin*	⚠	See description of point on page 234
Kidney Meridian				
Tai Xi	KID-3	Supreme Stream		
Zhao Hai	KID-6	Shining Sea		
Da He	KID-12	Great Luminance		Links with the Penetrating Vessel
Pericardium Meridian				
Nei Guan	PC-6	Inner Pass		Used for acupressure (pages 230–231)
Triple Burner Meridian (San Jiao)				
Yi Feng	TB-17	Wind Screen		Used for acupressure (pages 230–231)
Gall Bladder Meridian				
Feng Chi	GB-20	Wind Pool		Used for acupressure (pages 230–231)
Jian Jing	GB-21	Shoulder Well	⚠	Used for acupressure (pages 230–231)
Liver Meridian				
Tai Chong	LV-3	Great Rushing	⚠	
Extra points				
Yin Tang	EX-HN 3	Hall of Impression		See illustration of point on page 232
Tai Yang	EX-HN 5	Great Sun		Used for acupressure (pages 230–231)

	BLOOD STASIS	EXCESSIVE DAMP-HEAT	EXCESSIVE LIVER QI STAGNATION	EXCESSIVE PHLEGM-DAMP	COLD IN UTERUS	EXCESSIVE BLOOD HEAT	KIDNEY YIN DEFICIENCY	KIDNEY YANG DEFICIENCY	BLOOD AND QI DEFICIENCY
		✓							
	✓	✓	✓	✓	✓		✓	✓	✓
	✓		✓	✓	✓		✓	✓	✓
						✓			
						✓			
				✓					✓
		✓		✓					
			✓						
	✓	✓	✓	✓	✓		✓		✓
		✓		✓					
	✓					✓			
			✓			✓	✓		✓
			✓				✓		
				✓					
			✓	✓			✓		✓
				✓					
						✓	✓	✓	
					✓	✓	✓	✓	
								✓	
	✓		✓			✓			
			✓						

Chapter 3
TRADITIONAL CHINESE MEDICINE AND PREGNANCY

A couple's first visit to my clinic is often a time of anxiety and mixed feelings. Many have been trying unsuccessfully to become pregnant for a number of years. They may be tired, angry, sad, confused or desperate. Many people will have tried IVF (some several times) or may have tried using a donor egg or sperm and still not succeeded. They may have been told that they will not conceive at all or their chances of success are very slim.

My role (and the role of any TCM doctor) is to find out what is wrong in each individual case – why have they not been able to achieve a pregnancy, why assisted fertility treatment didn't work for them or why the pregnancy didn't go according to plan. I also need to identify their hopes and expectations and to support them in choosing the treatment that is right for them. In every circumstance it is very important to offer a realistic appraisal of their case, what we can do to help them, their chances of success and guide them in a direction that is right for them in terms of future fertility treatments.

Age is always a critical consideration. The average age at which women consult us is 37.8 years. Even though, at my clinic, we have helped a handful of women aged 46 to both conceive and achieve live births, the chances of success from age 45 onwards are greatly reduced. We have achieved a number of pregnancies in women aged 47 and over, but no live births so far. In spite of this evidence, some couples still want to try because they still have regular periods and reasonable ovarian reserves and they don't want to give up hope. They feel they need to give nature a chance and taking action provides hope. No matter what the statistics may indicate, some people still choose to try. As a practitioner it is important to be very patient. I try to help each person make a decision that is right for them – while respecting their right to choose their treatment.

People seek help at many different stages of the process and for many different reasons. Some come having already had surgical investigation or intervention, such as laparoscopy (a camera is inserted into the abdomen through a tiny hole to view the womb, fallopian tubes and ovaries). Others may have a polycystic ovary, which produces a lot of follicles but they don't mature into fertile eggs. Some may have tubal abnormalities, which cause mechanical problems, or endometriosis, which causes obstruction in the abdomen and needs to be cleared up to restore a normal blood supply to the ovaries and uterus, important for the ovaries to function normally and maximize the chances of implantation. Some of my patients are still young, but they may have low ovarian reserve, meaning the ovary is not functioning well and is behaving like the ovary of an older woman.

After taking a patient's history, the first questions I ask is, *'What would you like me to help you with*?' I know my patients come to me as they want to conceive, but some have already organized further IVF as they have been told that if they don't do it within the next few months they will run out of eggs. Most patients ask me what I think of their case and whether there is any hope.

There are two main elements to consider: the mechanical functioning of the woman's reproductive system, which may need investigation or surgical intervention; and reproductive health – the environment of the body, particularly the abdomen, which can be improved with the use of TCM. Often the two approaches will be combined, and some patients will opt for IVF in association with TCM. Other patients will not need IVF as 60 per cent of our pregnancies are conceived naturally.

Any form of assisted fertility treatment is very personal and the process can be an emotional journey. Everyone's needs are different and many people know themselves well enough to understand what is right for them. It is always the woman or the couple's decision. My role is to support and to be realistic, without destroying hope; to give them the chance I can offer and the help they need, while managing their expectations.

What is assisted fertility treatment?

Assisted fertility treatment includes: ovulation induction, Intra-Uterine Insemination (IUI), In-Vitro Fertilization (IVF) and Intra-Cytoplasmic Sperm Injection (ICSI). The most common assisted fertility treatment is In-Vitro Fertilization. In this method, instead of the sperm meeting and fertilizing the egg inside a woman's fallopian tube, the act of fertilization takes place outside the body. The woman's eggs are surgically removed using a fine needle passed into the ovaries. But because a woman usually only produces one egg each cycle, which would make IVF very unreliable, she is given drugs to stimulate her ovaries to produce more egg-bearing follicles, ideally around 15, the best of which are collected.

The man's sperm is collected and introduced to the eggs in a laboratory. The sperm will fertilize the eggs, creating embryos. Once the embryos are around two to three days old they will be transferred to the woman's womb. Previously, several embryos would be implanted to increase the chances of success, but too many IVF treatments were resulting in multiple births. These days just one or two are transferred because it is safer for the mother's health and gives the embryos a better chance of surviving to full term. If the woman is over 40, then sometimes three embryos may be transferred as she is deemed to be nearing the end of her productive life and her chances of trying again will be more limited.

Frozen Embryo Transfer (FET) Not all embryos created in the process of IVF are transferred to the uterus during IVF cycles. The ones that are not used can be frozen for use for an FET to produce a viable pregnancy at a later date. FET is likely to be used by couples who have been unsuccessful in becoming pregnant via other means, or by women who are over 46 years of age. There are a number of different FET protocols depending what is needed to appropriately prepare the uterus. Hence during an FET cycle, hormones may be introduced to the body to prompt the preparation of the uterine lining, or else the transfer may be performed using a natural cycle. The embryo is thawed and transferred to the uterus in the same way as during an IVF cycle.

ICSI (Intra-Cytoplasmic Sperm Injection) This can be used as part of the IVF procedure. During an ICSI cycle the best sperm is collected and injected directly into the egg, which gives the opportunity to select only the viable sperm. ICSI is frequently used when the man has a very low sperm count and where sperm motility is presenting difficulties. It is also used if the man has had a vasectomy, or where the woman has had problems relating to blocked tubes; or simply due to age. Sometimes the eggs are fragmentized and the sperm is unable to enter the egg to fertilize it.

IUI (Intra-Uterine Insemination) IUI is a procedure whereby the best-quality sperm are selected from a sample and prepared in a laboratory. They are then inserted into the womb at the woman's most fertile time, when an ovary releases an egg (ovulation).

IVF (In-Vitro Fertilization or 'test-tube') This is an assisted conception technique, which involves collecting the woman's egg and the man's sperm to fertilize them outside the body. The resulting early embryo is transferred into the cavity of the uterus.

Ovulation induction This technique usually uses fertility drugs to stimulate the follicles in the ovaries, resulting in the production of multiple eggs in one cycle. Some drugs also control the time that the eggs are released or when ovulation occurs, so sexual intercourse at a scheduled time will increase the chances of ovulation and achieving pregnancy.

What can go wrong?

Failure
IVF treatment does not always result in pregnancy. Currently around 20 to 25 per cent of IVF treatment cycles result in a birth. In general, younger women have a greater chance of success. Success rates decrease dramatically in women over 40.

Multiple pregnancy
There is an increased chance of multiple pregnancy through IVF. According to the British Fertility Society in September 2008, around 24 per cent of successful IVF cycles result in multiple births. Multiple pregnancy is associated with greater health risks for both mother and child as twins or triplets are more likely to be born prematurely and be underweight at birth.

Ovarian Hyper Stimulation Syndrome (OHSS)
Drugs used to stimulate the ovaries during IVF can lead to Ovarian Hyper Stimulation Syndrome (OHSS). In OHSS the ovaries enlarge and become painful, leading to abdominal discomfort. In more severe cases there can be shortness of breath, fluid retention in the abdominal cavity and formation of blood clots. In these cases OHSS can mean a stay in hospital.

Infection
When the eggs are harvested, a fine needle is passed through the vagina to the ovaries. There is a risk of introducing infection into the body, though antibiotics and surgical hygiene make this rare.

Emotional and psychological problems
IVF can be a stressful and emotionally demanding process for everyone. Some men and women suffer from anxiety or depression during or after IVF. Anyone undergoing IVF should be offered counselling to help with the emotional impact of the process and its result.

The benefits of choosing TCM

By the time my patients come to see me, almost all of them have tried some sort of assisted fertility treatment or are considering it. This is usually because couples who find they are not conceiving will go first to their GP, who will send them to the hospital for fertility testing. Before they know it they are being referred for assisted fertility treatment.

This would be fine if assisted fertility treatments were the magical answer to the problem. But in many cases they aren't. The success rate of the most common assisted fertility treatments is about 30 per cent for women below the age of 35. That means the failure rate is about 70 per cent. Many of the women who succeed could well have gone on to have babies naturally, and those who fail may give up trying for a baby altogether because of financial worries or physical and emotional stress. Often they are told by their consultant that they have very little time left to conceive as they are getting older; they are therefore encouraged to try one cycle of IVF after another.

At The Zhai Clinic, our statistics show that patients have, on average, failed four cycles of IVF before they come to us. That's a huge investment, both financially and emotionally.

Of course, there are many cases in which IVF is absolutely the right treatment and there are many successful pregnancies as a result. Overcoming blocked fallopian tubes, isolating individual sperm and increasing the number of eggs are all wonderful technological advances and I work very successfully with responsible assisted fertility clinics who, like me, are just trying to improve a couple's chance of conceiving.

But where I do feel that money is being wasted is when couples are told that assisted fertility treatment is the right way forward for them, despite the fact that other options haven't been explored. I have seen women in my clinic who have endured more than ten cycles of treatment without achieving a pregnancy, yet no one has stopped to ask whether something else is wrong, which should be treated before trying again.

For example, I treat many patients with polycystic ovaries, who can produce many follicles but all are of poor quality, with little chance of fertilization; I have seen patients who have recently undergone surgery to clear endometriosis who have been told to start IVF within a month of their operation, even though the blood flow to the abdomen is so poor the follicle-stimulating drugs couldn't possibly work. I once treated a woman who had undergone 18 cycles of IVF – imagine the toll that must have taken on her body and emotions, as well as her bank balance.

Responsible IVF consultants – and there are many – will always put the needs of the couple and the baby first but I do not doubt that there are some who continue to harvest follicles from women, despite knowing that many of those follicles will not produce a mature egg and that collecting them is a waste of time.

The stories I have included in this book are very typical of my patients and describe the kinds of health and infertility problems that have stood in the way of conception. The success stories are heart-warming and often a triumph of patience and commitment over the odds.

PART 2

TRADITIONAL CHINESE MEDICINE AND CONCEPTION

Chapter 4

DO YOU HAVE A FERTILITY PROBLEM?

Whether you are hoping to conceive in the future or have already made the life-changing decision to have a baby now, it's natural to want to become pregnant quickly – maybe as soon as you start trying. But just because your head has made a decision doesn't mean your body will follow suit. Getting pregnant may sound like a quick and natural process (and for many couples it is) but it's actually a complex interaction between a couple's constitution and genetic make-up, hormones, timing of the meeting between a good egg and progressive motile sperm, and a number of little glitches that may prevent fertilization.

It should not be at all surprising if you don't conceive immediately. After all, you may have spent years deliberately trying not to have a baby by using contraceptives, so why should your body be in such a hurry to become pregnant in the first few months? The delay doesn't automatically mean you are infertile. Everyone's body is different and will react in a different way with their partner's.

According to National Health Service (NHS) figures in the UK, for every 100 couples trying to conceive naturally:

- 20 will conceive within one month
- 70 will conceive within six months
- 85 will conceive within one year
- 90 will conceive within 18 months
- 95 will conceive within two years

But some people will have problems conceiving at all. In the UK it's thought to be as many as one in six or seven couples – that's around 3.5 million people. A couple is only diagnosed as infertile in the UK if they have not managed to conceive after having unprotected, regular sex for two years.

FERTILITY AND AGE

One of the most obvious things to bear in mind when planning a baby is that a woman's age is a significant factor in conception. However, it is eating healthily and keeping fit that will keep a woman's body in the best possible shape during its fertile lifespan.

- *In her 20s:* 10 out of 12 cycles may release eggs that are strong, good quality and ready for fertilization.

- *In her 30s:* 8 out of 12 cycles may release eggs that are good quality, strong and ready for fertilization; however, as age increases, egg quality and production declines.

- *In her early 40s:* there may be only 5 or 6 out of 12 cycles in which the egg quality is good enough for fertilization.

- *Over 44:* The egg quality and quantity will decline further. In my clinic, we have helped fewer than ten women aged 46 who have conceived with their own egg and gone on to achieve a live birth. I do know a woman (not my patient) who conceived at the age of 50 and gave birth to a healthy son when she was post-menopause. But cases like this are so rare they really are almost a miracle.

Case studies

Lucy is only 29 years of age; she met her husband ten years ago and had been on the contraceptive pill for ten years. She came off the pill less than six months ago and has been trying to get pregnant since. She is worried that she has a problem conceiving as she expected to conceive immediately (one of her friends got pregnant during the first month after she came off the pill). Her menstrual cycles are regular, she is young, fit and eats healthily.

When she came to see me I told her that if she was really worried I could organize some basic tests for her and her husband but I would rather that she relaxed more and tried not to think too much about getting pregnant each time she had sex. She should enjoy her life without contraception for at least a year or two before considering any tests or investigation. She should not worry about her fertility as she is young and it is normal for her not to have conceived yet – she may take up to two years.

Amanda, 35 years of age, has suffered from recurrent miscarriages in the past, but a course of Traditional Chinese Medicine (TCM) had helped her conceive. The pregnancy went to full term and she gave birth to healthy twins three years ago. She was a regular visitor to my clinic after the birth as she suffered from chronic arthritis for many years, with swollen and painful joints; TCM has helped relieve the pain and swollen joints. Amanda and her husband are having protected sex as she is not ready to conceive again yet. However, she would like to come back to see us when she is ready to try for a third baby.

Amanda has recurrent miscarriage history and general health problems. She is wise to use contraception to prevent pregnancy until she is ready as she does not want to risk another miscarriage. When she is ready to conceive, she can get TCM help before conception and afterwards to support her pregnancy.

Sara, 30, came off the pill after she and her husband got married. It took quite a long time for her periods to start again and they are irregular. For over a year they have been fluctuating from 50 to 70 days between periods.

Sara has absolutely every right to be concerned about her fertility and she needs to find out the reasons why her periods are so irregular. She should have all the necessary tests and investigations.

CLASSIFYING INFERTILITY

Once a couple has recognized that they have a fertility problem, they will generally be divided into two categories:

Primary infertility – where someone who has never achieved a pregnancy is having difficulty conceiving.

Secondary infertility – where a woman has had one or more pregnancies or babies in the past but is having difficulty conceiving again.

Couples in both these categories will need some sort of medical investigations to see what is preventing a pregnancy (see pages 79–81 and 83–85). But not all these couples will need to resort to assisted conception, such as IVF. Some may simply need to 'reboot' their bodies so that conception can take place naturally.

Whatever your reasons for needing to improve your fertility, it's important to be aware of how your own body functions before you can evaluate where the problem lies. That is why no treatment programme should begin without a thorough assessment of your current fertility health; and that applies to men as well as women.

The normal menstrual cycle

The complex interrelationship between hormones and timing necessary for successful fertilization relies on a healthy, regular menstrual cycle. Both Western medicine and

TCM agree that fertility is dependent on the release of hormones and that the pituitary gland in the brain controls hormone activity. The pituitary is only the size of a pea, but it controls the behaviour of many glands in the body, including the ovaries in women and the testes in men.

A woman's ovaries contain fluid-filled sacs, called follicles. At the beginning of each menstrual cycle, the hypothalamus area of the brain tells the pituitary gland to release follicle stimulating hormone (FSH). This hormone causes a number of the follicles in the ovaries to begin developing into an egg. Only one or two of these will actually mature each month and be released, ready to be fertilized.

Hormone activity also controls the preparation of a blood-rich, nutritious lining in the womb into which the egg can implant if it is fertilized. If fertilization does not occur, a drop in hormone levels causes the womb lining to be shed, and the cycle begins again with a menstrual bleed, or period.

This process is repeated during the course of each cycle throughout a woman's reproductive years, although the number of follicles reaching maturity will slowly fall as she ages. The length of the average menstrual cycle is 28 days, although it can be a couple of days less or more and still be a healthy cycle. The period of bleeding is, on average, five days. This monthly cycle is divided into two distinct parts, referred to as the follicular phase and the luteal phase; the change from one to the other is gradual.

USING FSH TO TREAT INFERTILITY

A common treatment for women who are having difficulty conceiving is to administer an injection of follicle stimulating hormone. However, this is not always successful. Some young women come to my clinic because they have not responded to the injection and none of their follicles has developed a mature egg.

I have found TCM can help. After TCM treatment, some women have gone on to achieve not only one pregnancy, but more. And those who are having IVF treatment may respond better to the drugs and produce more mature eggs than before. The healthy functioning of the reproductive system is the key. It is not simply that patients are running out of eggs so treatment with FSH isn't always successful.

THE FOLLICULAR PHASE

Day 1 of your cycle is the first day of your period; the day you start your menstrual bleed. The rise in FSH (see above) does exactly what the name suggests: it stimulates as many as 20 follicles in the ovary to grow, and as they ripen they release another hormone, oestrogen. When the level of oestrogen in the blood stream reaches a certain level, it causes the pituitary gland to stop producing FSH. At this point the most mature of the follicles goes on to release an egg; the less advanced follicles are simply reabsorbed by the body.

Around Day 12 or 13 of a 28-day cycle, the build-up of oestrogen produced by the maturing follicle triggers the pituitary gland to release luteinizing hormone (LH). The function of LH is to stimulate the follicle to release the mature egg into the fallopian tube. This process, called ovulation, usually takes place around Day 14, within 24 to 36 hours of the LH surge.

When the mature egg is released, the end of the fallopian tube gently takes hold of it. Here it may be fertilized by a sperm cell which has made the exhausting 'swim' up through the cervical mucus and the fallopian tube. The egg is viable for fertilization for about 24 to 36 hours after ovulation. However, depending on the exact time of ovulation, the flexibility of the fallopian tube and the travel time of the egg, conception could take place any time between Day 11 and Day 16, or even later. That is why I always advise my patients not to concentrate their efforts on a single day. They have a bigger window of opportunity than they may realize. For example, I once had a patient who didn't realize she was pregnant because her husband had been away during the ovulation period and they had not had intercourse until Day 17 of her cycle, yet that was the day on which she conceived.

Added to this, sperm can survive in a woman's body for up to three days before meeting and fertilizing an egg, which is why it is possible to become pregnant if you have intercourse before you have ovulated.

THE LUTEAL PHASE

The average length of the luteal phase is 14 days (between 10 and 16 days is considered normal). After ovulation, FSH and LH cause the now-empty egg follicle to transform itself into something called the corpus luteum. This secretes the hormone progesterone, which is essential for maintaining a pregnancy. Progesterone helps the endometrium (the lining of the womb) to become thick and rich in blood vessels, ready to receive the fertilized egg and provide it with nourishment from the mother's blood supply. It also causes the body's temperature to rise, something that is recorded on a BBT chart (see page 71).

If the egg is fertilized and successfully implants in the womb, this will trigger the production of the hormone human chorionic gonadotropin (HCG). This maintains the corpus luteum and ensures that it continues to produce progesterone to maintain the pregnancy. HCG is the hormone detected by pregnancy tests.

However, if the egg is not fertilized, the level of progesterone falls, which causes the womb to shed its thick lining. This is when your period starts, and is Day 1 of the next menstrual cycle.

The chart shows how levels of different hormones rise and fall in a typical 28-day cycle, where implantation and pregnancy do not take place.

Basal Body Temperature

Because an egg must be fertilized within 24 to 36 hours after being released by the ovary, knowing how your ovaries are functioning when you are ovulating and having sexual intercourse at the right time will significantly increase your chances of conceiving. Learning to read the signals your body gives off when it is about to ovulate is one of the most useful pieces of information you can have when trying for a baby.

Patients often come to me with the same question: *'All my blood tests are fine, all the investigations are fine, I don't have a problem with my fallopian tubes and my ultrasound scan shows that everything is in perfect order, why can't I conceive?'*

I suggest they start using a very basic method to monitor their cycle, the BBT chart, which shows how body temperature variations mirror hormonal changes during the monthly cycle. As you move through your menstrual cycle, your body temperature changes subtly as different hormones are produced to control the maturation and release of the egg.

Some fertility clinics aren't so keen on women monitoring their own temperatures, as they feel it is time-consuming when they have more scientific methods available. Many Western fertility doctors regard BBT charts as outdated in the technological world, believing that they simply add stress to the routine of a childless couple. My view is that the temperature chart is not just about ovulation: it is the simplest, cheapest and, indeed, the only way to understand your own body and how your ovaries are functioning.

Learning to read the fluctuations in your own cycle allows you to understand why your body isn't getting pregnant, even if you are ovulating every month, and also allows you to monitor your progress, as the TCM gradually improves your natural fertility cycle. I think it is an extremely important and effective tool.

It takes only a couple of minutes each day to take your temperature and chart it. I find that rather than being a chore, for many of my patients this is a fascinating insight into what is happening to their bodies. After all, what's a few minutes every day for a few months when it could dramatically improve your chances of getting pregnant?

Of course, I also understand that being unable to conceive can be very distressing and draining but I believe the light this daily monitoring shines on your fertility will outweigh any negative emotions it creates.

BBT charting involves no equipment apart from a thermometer, pen and paper yet it reveals a mass of information about your hormones and menstrual cycle, including the length of the cycle and the days on which intermenstrual, postmenstrual or premenstrual bleeding or spotting occurs. Keeping a chart can also reveal whether you are having reasonably regular sexual intercourse.

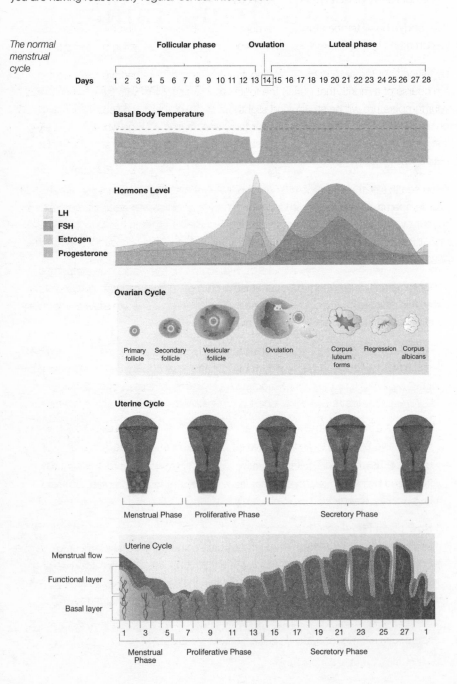

The normal menstrual cycle

Follicular phase **Ovulation** **Luteal phase**

Days 1 2 3 4 5 6 7 8 9 10 11 12 13 14 15 16 17 18 19 20 21 22 23 24 25 26 27 28

Basal Body Temperature

Hormone Level

LH
FSH
Estrogen
Progesterone

Ovarian Cycle

Primary follicle · Secondary follicle · Vesicular follicle · Ovulation · Corpus luteum forms · Regression · Corpus albicans

Uterine Cycle

Menstrual Phase · Proliferative Phase · Secretory Phase

Uterine Cycle

Menstrual flow
Functional layer
Basal layer

1 3 5 7 9 11 13 15 17 19 21 23 25 27 1

Menstrual Phase · Proliferative Phase · Secretory Phase

STARTING A CHART

I recommend buying a special digital BBT fertility thermometer, because it is much easier to read first thing in the morning. A few months of consistent BBT charts can often tell your fertility status; any patient who comes to me for treatment will know that joining those dots every day can draw a very accurate picture of their fertility profile.

Your body's basal temperature is your normal daily temperature first thing in the morning. I recommend that you take it as soon as you wake up, before getting out of bed.

By taking your temperature and plotting it every day on your chart, you will see over the course of a month that during the follicular phase of your cycle (see pages 65–66), your temperature will be steady and slightly lower than during the second or luteal phase of your cycle (see page 66). Your temperature may change when you ovulate; first there may be a brief drop, then a slow rise. Many women don't see the fall but notice when their temperature begins to rise, which is equally good.

If you see this pattern emerge over a couple of months you will learn, for example, that your temperature drops quickly, then slowly begins to rise again around Days 12 to 14 of your cycle if you have a 28-day cycle. This indicates ovulation has taken place and that you should ideally be having sex not only at this time but also ideally two or three days before and two or three days after too.

If your temperature stays elevated for at least 12 days during the luteal phase of your cycle, this indicates that enough progesterone is being produced to allow the fertilized egg to successfully implant in the lining of the womb.

PLANNING SEXUAL INTERCOURSE

Many of my patients admit that they find planned sexual intercourse becomes hard work. Men find it difficult to perform at a particular time so having sex becomes a job rather than a pleasure. Most of my patients are not failing to conceive because they don't have enough sexual intercourse. Instead, because they find it difficult to conceive, they start trying too hard and become frustrated by performing to a timetable. As months pass by, they find it more and more difficult to perform.

How often should we have sex?

I ask my patients how often they normally have intercourse, and tell them to mark on their BBT chart each time it occurs. I tell them to carry on doing what they normally do, and not to have sex just because they want to show me they have not missed their ovulation. The theory is that if couples have intercourse twice a week (every three days), they will never miss the fertile period as healthy sperm can survive for up to 72 hours in a woman's body.

I am particularly against the idea of having sex every day around the time of ovulation, partly because it can create emotional tension as I mentioned before, but also I believe it can put pressure on the fine fallopian tubes, which help the egg travel towards the womb.

Daily sex can also reduce sperm quality: there will be fewer fast-moving, motile sperm to fertilize the egg. Men with a low sperm count would be best advised to save up sperm for use on the day of ovulation, or one or two days before.

Case studies

Margaret is 43; she has been trying to conceive her second child for the last four years. She has a regular 28-day cycle and her fertility condition has much improved over the last few months of TCM treatment. One day, Margaret turned up for her follow-up consultation and was terribly upset. She had missed her ovulation this cycle as her husband was away and hadn't come home until Day 17 of her cycle. However, we discovered she had conceived during this cycle – why?

She had been concentrating so hard on getting everything right for conception, including the timing. She assumed that she could not become pregnant during this cycle because her ovulation date had passed. But because she was not thinking about it too much and was relaxed, conception happened naturally.

Leona was 41 when she came to see me after three failed IVF cycles. One of her fallopian tubes had been removed as a result of an ectopic pregnancy from the IVF. She told me that if I was able to help her, that would be great but she was not planning any further assisted fertility treatment.

After eight months of TCM treatment, I told Leona and her husband that Leona was ready and a pregnancy could happen any time. However, every cycle when her period started, she came to see me with her eyes swollen and I knew that she had been crying.

One year and three months into the TCM treatment, Leona's family visited them from abroad. The couple were so busy taking them sightseeing, even travelling back to her home town with them, that she was surprised to find she was pregnant. And she couldn't even remember when they had had sexual intercourse. Why hadn't conception happened sooner? She was ready to conceive, but the tension and high expectations had prevented it.

The chart (see opposite) is an example of a cycle that is working well. Perhaps the patient needs only to adjust the timing of her sexual activity or improve the blood flow to her womb to help implantation. But many patients' charts reveal underlying problems, or simply that a patient's cycle doesn't conform to the norm.

Name																																			
Month																	September/October																		
Date	14	15	16	17	18	19	20	21	22	23	24	25	26	27	28	29	30	1	2	3	4	5	6	7	8	9	10	11	12						
Day of cycle	1	2	3	4	5	6	7	8	9	10	11	12	13	14	15	16	17	18	19	20	21	22	23	24	25	26	27	28	29	30	31	32	33	34	35
38.2																																			
38.1																																			
38.0																																			
37.9																																			
37.8																																			
37.7																																			
37.6																																			
37.5																																			
37.4																																			
37.3																																			
37.2																																			
37.1																				•															
37.0																•			•																
36.9														•			•	•			•		•												
36.8																						•													
36.7															•																				
36.6																								•											
36.5																									•	•									
36.4	•						•		•		•	•																•							
36.3		•	•		•			•		•																				Commence New Chart					
36.2				•		•																													
36.1																																			
36.0													•																						
35.9																																			
35.8																																			
35.7																																			
35.6																																			
35.5																																			
Bleeding	X	X	X	X	X																						X	X	X						
Intercourse						X		X		X	X	X		X				X																	

This is an ideal temperature chart. The cycle is 28 days; the first half of the cycle (the follicular phase) shows a relatively low and steady temperature, which indicates follicles growing in an uninterrupted and healthy manner. During the second part of the cycle (the luteal phase), the temperature is confidently and consistently raised, which shows that there is no problem with ovulation, and also indicates the progesterone level would be sufficient to support a fertilized egg.

It's possible that your chart will not show this typically healthy pattern but with TCM treatment you can hope to achieve a chart close to this example.

When a woman has achieved a healthy chart consistently for three cycles, together with a good pulse reading, tongue texture and colour, it is a sign that her body is in a receptive condition and this is the time that she should try to relax as she is ready to conceive.

COMPILING A CHART

Copy the chart shown here or use a chart supplied by your doctor. Start a new chart as soon as your period starts, as this is Day 1 of your cycle. Mark the calendar date on the chart.

1. Before you go to bed each evening, place your clean thermometer on the bedside table. A digital BBT thermometer is easiest to use but if you have a glass mercury thermometer make sure you have shaken it down to below 36°C. Use the same thermometer, preferably at a similar time each morning, throughout the months you are keeping your chart.

2. Before you get up each morning, put the thermometer under your tongue, and leave it in place for at least 5 minutes if you are using a mercury thermometer, or 1 minute if you are using a digital thermometer.

3. Remove and read the thermometer carefully.

4. Record your temperature for each day, by marking a dot on the chart at the temperature indicated on the thermometer. As the days pass, join the dots by marking a straight line between dots for adjacent days.

5. Mark any other relevant information on the chart beside the dot, such as whether you had a disturbed night, if you have a cold, a sore throat or an attack of indigestion. You should also record on which days bleeding occurs, and on which days you have sexual intercourse.

The information you have recorded can be used to see the length of your cycle, your days of bleeding, the frequency of intercourse and the date of ovulation. You can even add the results of ovulation prediction tests if you wish to use them as well (see below).

OVULATION PREDICTORS

Some of my patients ask why we use temperature charts when ovulation predictor kits are available. Ovulation predictors test your urine on specific days of your cycle to detect a high level of luteinizing hormone, which triggers ovulation.

However, they are not necessarily accurate if you have irregular periods or another health issue such as Polycystic Ovary Syndrome (PCOS). I have found that many women who do ovulate regularly still have problems getting pregnant, so ovulation is only part of the jigsaw. You may be ovulating well, but your luteal phase temperature may drop, which reflects a malfunction of the reproductive system, something an ovulation predictor will not show. Ovulation predictors cannot prove whether your ovaries are in good form either.

So I believe ovulation predictors can suggest when it is the best time to have intercourse, but they cannot offer the rest of the information that a BBT chart can, plus they are expensive. My advice for a healthy couple is that, provided you have intercourse twice a week, you will never miss your most fertile period.

Case studies

Sawtooth pattern and insufficient temperature rise

Rowena was a 39-year-old business consultant. She had come to us when trying to conceive her first child and was diagnosed with polycystic ovaries. We treated her with TCM for three months and she had then conceived naturally and given birth to a son. Since that time, she had been trying to conceive again; but over a year had passed with no success.

She complained of premenstrual tension and heavy menstrual bleeding with a few clots. She also suffered from constipation and disturbed sleep, sometimes feeling hot at night.

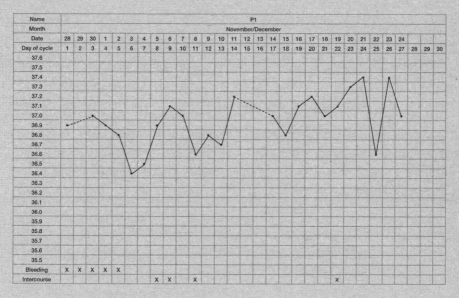

Figure 1 – This chart shows a sawtooth pattern.

Rowena's temperature charts (Figures 1 and 2) show a sawtooth pattern with a number of high peaks. With this kind of wide, unexplained temperature oscillation in the follicular phase, Liver Heat must be suspected and, in particular with a pre-ovulation temperature of between 36.5°C and 37.1°C, also Blood Heat. Constipation is typically a symptom of Heat. The instability in the luteal phase points to Liver *qi* stagnation.

The change in Basal Body Temperature across the cycle was so insignificant that it suggested to me either a deficiency of both *yin* and *yang*; or possibly insufficient *yin* to provide the basis for *yang* to rise. This insufficiency of *yin* is also reflected in Rowena's symptom of sometimes feeling hot at night. When this pattern shows in the BBT chart, I prescribe a more regular lifestyle with less stress and a relaxation regime to complement treatment.

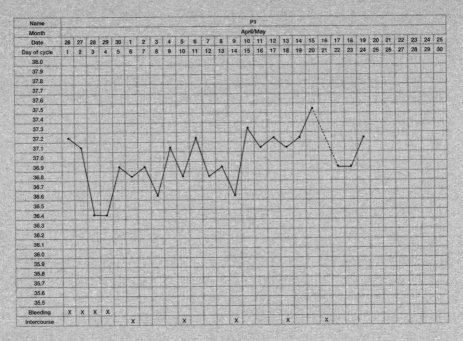

Figure 2 – Here a slight temperature rise occurs in the luteal phase.

In both Figures 1 and 2, the temperature rise during the luteal phase is only slight (36.4°C to 37.5°C). In TCM a luteal phase of just nine or ten days suggests Spleen *qi* deficiency and mild Kidney weakness. This can compromise fertility because there is insufficient time for the follicle to implant properly. Rowena's disturbed sleep also suggested *qi* and Blood deficiency.

In Rowena's case, TCM treatment was focused initially on soothing Liver stagnation and cooling the Blood Heat. Next we focused on tonifying the Kidney *yin*. And then Rowena became pregnant again.

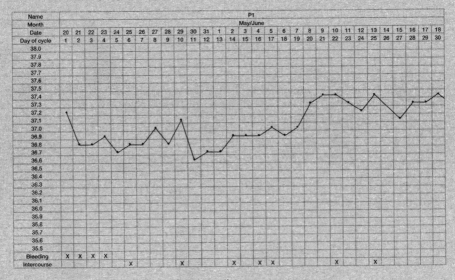

Figure 3 – Improved luteal phase, showing conception.

Figure 3 shows that Rowena's follicular phase improved during the course of her TCM treatment and that conception was achieved. This can be seen by a luteal phase with raised temperature after Day 18, but with no bleeding. However, the luteal phase was unstable. For example, on Day 27 of the cycle, and Day 39 (not shown), the 0.2°C temperature drop suggests that Spleen *qi* and the Kidney may not yet be strong enough to support firm implantation. When BBT is notably unstable during the months prior to pregnancy, care must be taken as there is a greater likelihood of miscarriage.

A lengthened follicular phase and irregular cycle

Nicola was 36 years old when she came to see us. She and her husband had not used contraception for three years and had been trying to conceive for the last two and a half years. They underwent three Intra-Uterine Insemination (IUI) cycles with ovulation induction and one IVF cycle. During the second IUI cycle, Nicola did conceive but the embryo stopped growing very early on, before it was large enough to be seen by ultrasound. This, known as a biochemical pregnancy, is in effect a very early form of miscarriage – potentially triggered by chromosomal abnormalities.

Nicola had had a pelvic ultrasound scan a year earlier, which indicated her ovary had a polycystic appearance, though the hysteroscopy, HSG and hormone tests showed no abnormalities. Her cycle was 30 to 46 days long, with four or five days of bleeding. She had recently developed a lot of acne on her face.

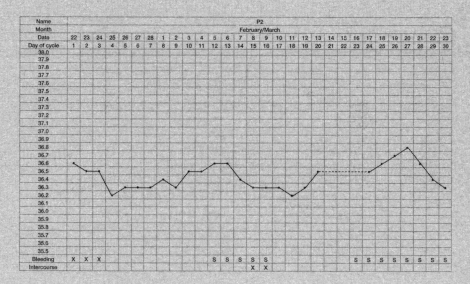

Figure 1 – Ovulation occurs on Day 18.

A lengthened follicular phase within an irregular cycle is typically seen in patients with polycystic ovaries (see pages 91–92). Their ovaries are likely to be enlarged because they contain excessive fluids, so they can't receive the healthy blood necessary to nourish and support follicle growth. The follicles are therefore unable to mature and natural ovulation may be delayed or difficult. In TCM this extended follicular phase can be interpreted as showing an insufficiency of Kidney essence, *yin* and Blood; or due to *qi* stagnation obstructing ovulation.

Polycystic ovaries can disrupt the blood supply to the uterus, so the lining takes a longer time to form. Although the temperatures for Days 21 to 23 of the cycle are missing in Figure 1, the chart shows an unstable luteal phase (also confirmed in Figure 2). From a TCM perspective it indicates stagnation of Liver *qi*.

Nicola also presented with spotting between Days 12 to 16 and Days 23 to 30 of her cycle. Abnormal bleeding patterns in ovulatory cycles are often unexplained, though may be due to an insufficient luteal phase. Mid-cycle spotting probably indicates that the growth and structure of the womb lining has not been established soundly in the follicular phase, which points towards an oestrogen deficiency, related in TCM to *yin* and Blood deficiency or too much Heat. Nicola also had premenstrual spotting, which is related to incomplete breakdown of the corpus luteum and is associated in TCM with Blood stasis.

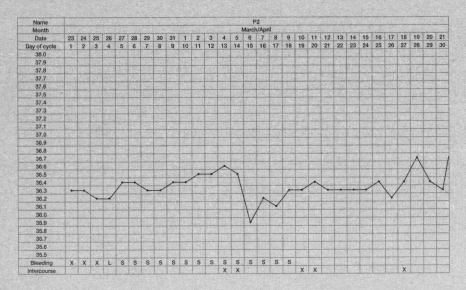

Figure 2 – Ovulation occurs on Day 26.

Figure 2 shows that a temperature dip is recorded on Day 15 of Nicola's cycle. However, the temperature rise that follows is insufficient to suggest that ovulation has occurred. On Day 26 of the cycle, another dip is recorded followed by a temperature rise of at least 0.2°C above the *highest* of the six preceding lowest values. This suggests ovulation. Nicola had a frozen embryo transfer (FET) on Day 26 but, sadly for her, it was unsuccessful.

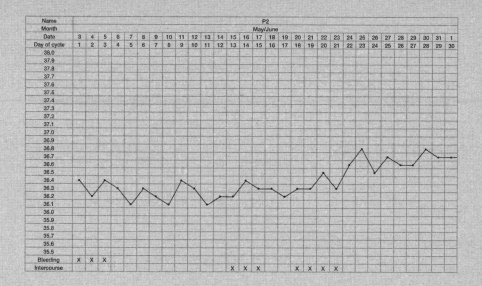

Figure 3 – Luteal phase with raised temperature after Day 18, with no bleeding, suggesting pregnancy.

The purpose of the TCM treatment in Nicola's case was to clear her abdominal obstruction, which was formed by excessive fluids, and to get her blood flowing more freely so that her blood supply was able to circulate to her abdomen and ovaries.

There was a positive result for Nicola during the next cycle when she achieved a spontaneous pregnancy. Figure 3 shows normal blood loss during her period. Her Blood stasis had been resolved satisfactorily. She bled normally for three days with good flow, without any spotting, and managed to achieve pregnancy very early on in her normal cycle.

Stabilization of the luteal phase

Cara was a 37-year-old nurse who already had one child, a daughter of 12. She had been trying to conceive again for the last five years, but had been unsuccessful, apart from one pregnancy which resulted in an early miscarriage four years ago.

Her cycles were slightly prolonged, varying between 28 and 40 days (although most were 31 days). She complained of headaches before her periods and a slightly bloated stomach. Her tongue was dry, with no coating. Her prolonged menstrual cycles indicated a Blood deficiency, while her headaches and bloated stomach indicated that she had Liver *qi* stagnation. The TCM treatment we gave Cara was designed to improve Blood flow and sooth Liver *qi*.

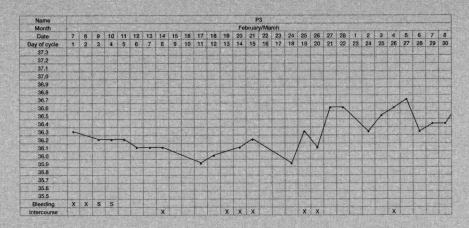

Figure 1 – This shows insignificant ovulation and an erratic luteal phase.

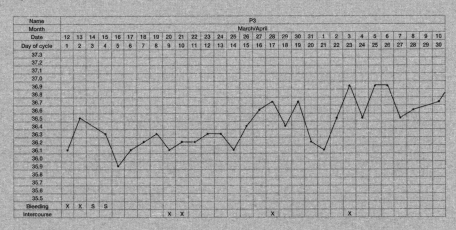

Figure 2 – This show ovulation on Day 14 and a stabilization of the cycle from Day 27 on.

Figure 2 shows that Cara ovulated on Day 14 of her cycle. Her luteal phase was a little erratic, perhaps due to the shifts she was working, but it became very stable from Day 27. Her BBT continued to rise steadily and a pregnancy was confirmed.

WHEN TO SEEK HELP

If you are under 35, have been trying to get pregnant with no success for two years, are having sex at least twice a week (not just at weekends) and have no other obvious health problems, it is time to consult a doctor whether your temperature chart appears normal or not.

Your first visit, as a couple, should be to your family doctor, who will ask you a series of questions about your menstrual cycle, health history and sexual intercourse habits.

You will probably be a little anxious on your first visit, whether to a Western or TCM doctor, but remember to take some basic information with you (write it down if you become tongue-tied in the surgery!) such as: the age you started your periods, the length of your cycle and whether your periods are regular, how heavy they are and how painful they are. See pages 251–258 for a complete list of the questions I ask my patients.

Your doctor might do a physical examination and will also probably suggest some basic tests, which could reveal where your problem lies. The following section explains what to expect.

Tests for women

These are the fertility tests a family doctor might suggest for a woman.

BLOOD HORMONE TESTS

Some basic blood tests can help diagnose hormonal imbalances that may affect your ability to conceive. The tests measure levels of FSH, LH, oestrogen and prolactin in the blood and need to be performed at the beginning of the menstrual cycle, between Day 1 and Day 5, ideally on Day 3. If the level of LH is high at the beginning of the cycle, this may prevent the necessary surge around the time of ovulation and may also indicate Polycystic Ovary Syndrome (PCOS). Prolactin is a 'stress' hormone and high levels in the blood could prevent the release of FSH and LH, and can occasionally reveal a problem with the pituitary gland.

In recent years, the Anti-Mullerian hormone test has become commonly used as an indicator of a woman's ovarian condition. This test is considered to be very effective in detecting conditions that can be contributing to a delay in getting pregnant. This test is also performed on Day 3 of the cycle.

It is normal practice for a family doctor to measure progesterone levels in your blood on Day 21 of a normal 28-day cycle too. However, I rarely do this myself as I find most of the women I treat have a sufficient progesterone level and their BBT chart will show whether or not the level is within the normal range.

ULTRASOUND SCANNING

An ultrasound scan can be used to check the development of the follicle, the thickness of the womb lining and if and when ovulation occurs. It may also reveal the presence of fibroids in the womb or ovarian cysts. Ultrasound scanning is also used during pregnancy to evaluate the health of a growing foetus.

TUBAL PATENCY TESTS

These tests check whether or not your fallopian tubes are fully open. Clear, healthy fallopian tubes will allow the ascending sperm free passage to reach the egg, and a fertilized egg free passage to reach the uterus for implantation. It is quite rare for a blocked fallopian tube to show any external symptoms so you will probably be unaware of the condition and this routine test will be one of the first things your doctor prescribes.

The most common cause of blocked or damaged fallopian tubes is a previous infection that may have gone untreated or unnoticed. Pelvic Inflammatory Disease (PID) is the most common of these. Sexually transmitted diseases such as chlamydia or gonorrhoea can also cause damage so it's important to tell your doctor if you have ever suffered from any of these conditions.

If you have had a surgical procedure for miscarriage or abortion in the past, these may have affected your fallopian tubes so, again, do tell your doctor. Another possible cause of blocked tubes is a ruptured appendix or abdominal surgery.

HYSTEROSALPINGOGRAM (HSG)

This test can evaluate whether your fallopian tubes and uterus have any structural abnormalities and whether a pregnancy will occur naturally. Radiographic contrast fluid (dye) is injected into the uterine cavity (womb) through a narrow catheter inside the vagina and cervix. The uterine cavity fills with dye and if the fallopian tubes are open, dye fills the tubes and spills out into the abdominal cavity. The test is performed between Day 7 and Day 10 of your menstrual cycle and it is very important that you are not pregnant at the time the test is performed.

HYSTEROSALPINGO-CONTRAST-SONOGRAPH (HYCOSY)

This test is similar to an HSG but uses ultrasound technology. It is normally carried out between Day 8 and Day 10 of your cycle. Echo contrast fluid (dye) is injected into the uterine cavity (womb) through a narrow catheter inside the vagina and cervix. An ultrasound scanning head is inserted into the vagina to view the ovaries and check that the fallopian tubes are clear and the uterine cavity is free of fibroids or cysts.

HYSTEROSCOPY

A hysteroscopy is a procedure used to examine the inside of the uterus (womb). It is normally carried out by using a narrow tube with a hysteroscope (a kind of small telescope) at the end. Images are sent to a computer to give a close-up image of the womb. This procedure can be used to help diagnosis in cases where a woman's symptoms suggest that there may be a problem with the womb, such as recurrent miscarriage, heavy or irregular periods, pelvic pain, unusual discharge or bleeding between periods. A hysteroscopy can also be used to identify abnormal growths from the womb, including fibroids, polyps and intra-uterine adhesions.

LAPAROSCOPY

A laparoscopy is a keyhole surgical procedure that allows access to the inside of the abdomen and the pelvis. A small incision is made just below the navel, through which is inserted a small flexible tube containing a light and a camera (a laparoscope). The camera relays images of the inside of the abdomen or pelvis to a screen.

The procedure is used to help diagnose a wide range of conditions that develop inside the abdomen or pelvis, including adhesions from endometriosis, Pelvic Inflammatory Disease (PID) or fibroids. It can also be used to carry out surgical procedures such as laser treatment or diathermy to remove adhesions and mobilize the ovary after fertilization.

Case study

Georgia, aged 42

PROBLEM:	**raised FSH levels, endometriosis and tubal hydrosalpinx**
METHODS TRIED:	**3 IVF cycles**
TCM OBJECTIVE:	**to clear the Heat and Damp, soothe the Liver and improve Kidney *yin***
LENGTH OF TREATMENT:	**10 months for the first pregnancy; 6 months for the second**
OUTCOME:	**natural conception; 2 children in the long term**

Georgia came to see us after three failed IVF attempts, having tried two fertility clinics. On each occasion the IVF cycles were abandoned. Either the follicles were too small, or there were too few, or she ovulated before egg collection. She had developed a high fever during two attempts, while being on FSH injections. She sought the opinion of another consultant but the option on offer was to try a further IVF cycle, perhaps using a different fertility drug. Having read an article about us in a magazine, she decided it was time to try TCM, and a different approach.

TCM assessment
Georgia had not had any fertility investigations apart from some hormone tests. Her FSH levels were raised, between 12 and 26, and so I told Georgia that further IVF would be very difficult as her ovaries were tired and she would not respond well to the FSH injection.

Georgia was only 42 years old; she seemed healthy apart from some endometriosis, which had been diagnosed some years before and which may have put pressure on her ovaries. They were having to work hard, were not motile and were unable to perform, which was reflected in both the quality and quantity of eggs.

Georgia wanted an alternative option, other than IVF. I invited her to take a Hysterosalpingo-Contrast-Sonograph (HYCOSY) to check the viability of the fallopian tubes, to see whether she was capable of conceiving by herself. The test revealed Georgia had hydrosalpinx (a fallopian tube blocked at its outer end), which it was thought could cause some fluid to be retained in the fallopian tube. This may prevent conception or implantation, or else cause the fluid to get to the uterus and cause damage to the embryo – which could also compromise implantation.

Yet another fertility specialist then recommended a further round of IVF as being her most suitable option. The consultant further explained to her that her damaged fallopian tubes needed to be surgically removed even if Georgia didn't want IVF. Georgia was completely devastated. She said she felt as if she was walking through a dark tunnel, unable to see the light. Desperate for a sign of hope, she consulted a leading IVF specialist in New York who believed the results were inconclusive. He suggested Georgia continue with TCM treatment.

TCM treatment plan

The endometriosis and hydrosalpinx made clearing the abdominal obstruction the first priority. We worked on clearing the Damp and Heat in the abdominal environment to get the blood flow going. Once this was established, I worked on improving her internal organs, particularly improving the Kidney *yin* to support the ovary function. The treatment changed all the time according to her response and progression. Her hot flashes and peri-menopausal symptoms reduced, but her FSH levels remained high. At our recommendation, Georgia increased her exercise levels and improved her nutrition and diet. During her six months of TCM treatment, Georgia's general health improved a great deal and her menstrual cycles became more regular.

A further two months into her treatment Georgia said to me, *'Dr Zhai I have a feeling I do not need IVF. I think I can do it myself.'* And that is exactly what happened. Ten months into treatment, she conceived.

I was amazed by the outcome – but this is not the only time it has happened. I do think that many patients have a deep understanding of what they need – sometimes more than the fertility experts. The patient knows her body – and sometimes she knows how she feels and whether she is up to getting pregnant or not. The herbs, too, have a powerful effect on the body and encourage people to become more in tune with their body's health and enable a sense of wellbeing and balance.

A word about FSH

Hormones are produced by endocrine glands and some of these hormones control the normal functioning of women's reproductive organs. One of the glands, the pituitary, releases a hormone called follicle stimulating hormone (FSH).

FSH travels via the blood to the ovaries where it stimulates a follicle or group of follicles to start to grow and develop. It is inside these follicles that the eggs begin to develop – one in each follicle. As the follicles grow, the follicle cells begin to release another hormone called oestrogen. Oestrogen travels up to the brain to block further release of FSH from the pituitary. This is called feedback inhibition.

The FSH (follicle stimulating hormone) level is a measure of a woman's ovarian reserve – that means the ability of the ovary to produce viable eggs for fertilization. Normal levels are within the range of approximately 2–12 mIU/ml. For a woman who is trying to conceive, the lower the result the better, because that means the ovaries are not having to work too hard.

A lot of people come to me and say, 'My FSH level is really high, can you help me to lower it?' I have to say that it doesn't really work that way. FSH is a measure of how hard your ovaries are working. The focus should not be on lowering the FSH level, but improving your ovary function. If the ovary is functioning within the normal range, then it does not need much FSH to induce a follicle to develop and the level will be within normal range.

An elevated level of FSH is one of the most common conditions affecting women who are finding it difficult to conceive. Often, these women find that they are turned away from fertility clinics because they generally respond very poorly, if at all, to the drugs used to stimulate their ovaries for IVF treatment. If by chance they do respond, the egg quality is usually poor and numbers are very few. Many fertility specialists consider that it is not possible to reverse this condition and would advise women to consider using donor eggs. However, it can be hard to come to terms with the idea of using donor eggs, and most women prefer to be able to have their own genetically related child if at all possible. TCM treatment may give some hope to some of those women.

Tests for men

Semen analysis is the basic test of male fertility. This test can be arranged by your family doctor, and you are advised to have at least two semen analyses.

A semen analysis is an important tool for the early diagnosis of male fertility problems, to diagnose the extent of infertility and to ensure appropriate treatment. It can also sometimes prevent unnecessary investigation of the woman, which can save valuable time if the woman's age is an issue.

However, clinics and hospitals use different criteria when assessing the sperm and the results could vary. You must also be aware that some assisted fertility clinics may only test whether the sperm sample is good enough for IUI, IVF or ICSI. They may not advise whether the sperm is good enough for natural conception.

WHAT DOES SEMEN ANALYSIS INVOLVE?

The man will be asked to produce a sample of sperm to be examined in a laboratory. Because the sperm should be as fresh as possible, it's advisable to actually produce the sample at the hospital or laboratory where it will be tested. Specimens may be produced at home only if they can reach the laboratory within 30 minutes and, in these circumstances, the laboratory will give you instructions on what to do. Samples that do not arrive at the laboratory within the required time will produce unreliable and misleading results.

Normally, the laboratory will advise patients to abstain from ejaculation for three days before producing the specimen for assessment. They will advise that it is essential that patients do not abstain for longer than five days, or fewer than two days (three days in the case of DNA fragmentation, see box, below), otherwise the quantity of sperm will be affected. In my view, however, if you have a low sperm count or low motility, you could abstain a little longer to see whether this produces a better sample, particularly if it needs to be used for IVF or ICSI.

SPERM DNA FRAGMENTATION

The sperm cell contains long strands of genetic material, DNA, that are tightly packed together, rather like a ball of yarn. It is designed for fast and flexible movement. Unlike other cells in the body, sperm are unable to repair themselves when damaged because they lack the enzymes necessary, so they are susceptible to damage and the DNA strands may become broken. This is known as DNA fragmentation. An egg that is fertilized by a fragmented sperm is unlikely to go to full term.

WHAT CAN A SPERM SAMPLE TELL US?

Your doctor will be looking at the number of sperm in the sample, its appearance, its motility (how well it 'swims') and the quality of it.

According to the latest World Health Organization report:

- A low sperm count is below 15 million per millilitre (ml) of semen.
- Motility means that at least 40 per cent of the sperm are motile with a forward progression rate of 32 per cent, or 2+ on the scale of 0–4 (see box, opposite).

- Poor motility means that less than 40 per cent of sperm are motile and fewer than 32 per cent of sperm have a progression rate of 2+.
- Poor sperm quality means low motility and/or a high proportion of abnormal forms of sperm (more than 96%), for example, displaying chromosomal abnormality.

There are also criteria for measuring and assessing the shape and size of the sperm (known as the morphology) but it is difficult to predict pregnancy based on this detail.

SPERM MOTILITY CHART

0	No movement
1	Movement, none forward
1+	Occasional movement of a few sperm
2	Slow; undirected movement
2+	Slow; directly forward movement
3-	Fast; undirected movement
3	Fast; directly forward movement
3+	Very fast forward movement
4	Extremely fast forward movement

TREATMENTS FOR MALE INFERTILITY

In Western medicine, most men diagnosed with a poor sperm count or quality will be advised to use Intra-Cytoplasmic Sperm Injection (ICSI) treatment as Western medicine offers no other way to overcome a man's infertility problems (although he may have been advised to keep his testicles cool by avoiding hot baths and wearing pure cotton underwear, or to stop cycling). In TCM, poor sperm count or quality can be effectively treated using a combination of herbs and acupuncture.

However, when a couple comes to me for help, I analyse the woman's reproductive health first and treat any problems before I treat the man's problem. My results show that until a woman's reproductive health is in optimum condition, there will be no pregnancy, even if the man's semen sample is very good quality. See pages 98–101 for more about male fertility problems.

Case study

Philip and **Karen**, both in their early 40s, had been trying to conceive for two years before resorting to fertility investigation and treatment. The obvious problem was that Philip has a very low sperm count (less than 1 million per ml) and his most recent sample contained just 20 motile sperm in all. The couple had failed to conceive on their first two ICSI cycles and were planning for a third attempt.

The clinic the couple attended told them that the failure was due to Philip's low sperm count: the clinic had only a few sperm to choose from. So Philip and Karen came to me to improve the semen sample before undergoing the next ICSI treatment.

However, I wanted to check out Karen too, as I thought that although she was all clear in the mechanical/anatomical aspects of her fertility, she may have a low reserve of poor-quality eggs, due to her age. This was confirmed and accounted for the fact that during each of her last ICSI cycles she produced only a few follicles and just one of the three eggs was fertilized, which was of poor quality. So it wasn't just a low sperm count but also the poor quantity and quality of Karen's eggs that was preventing conception.

I treated them both with TCM. By the second month of Philip's treatment, his sperm count improved to 80 million per ml but the motility was still low, at 14 per cent. The IVF clinic, and the couple themselves, were so surprised by the improvement in Philip's sperm count they suspected that the sample must have been mixed up with that of another patient. By Philip's third month of TCM treatment, although the sperm count was less, at 45 million per ml, the motility had improved to 40 per cent. This was the more important factor. After several months of treating Karen, she became pregnant. Not as an outcome of ICSI, but naturally.

Chapter 5

CAUSES OF INFERTILITY

Most of the couples I see in my clinic believe, or have been told, that they have a fertility problem that the assisted fertility clinic is unable to help with. Some of them will have had preliminary or extensive tests; some of them will have failed many assisted fertility treatments. In the past, I saw only women who had tried all the available treatments unsuccessfully and were trying TCM as a final option, before giving up their desire to have their own baby or move on to the donor eggs programme. In more recent years, many people come to the clinic simply because they have been unable to conceive naturally and want help. There is more awareness of the fertility options available now, and more people are choosing TCM as their first option. With all my patients I approach the problem in a similar way.

My methods are a unique blend of Western medical diagnostic techniques and TCM, so I use the best each system has to offer to determine what the problem is, what treatment (if any) is best for the patients and when would be the best time to try a cycle of assisted fertility treatment, if necessary.

Western diagnostic and fertility treatment techniques are invaluable in cases that need surgical intervention and where there is a physical problem preventing patients conceiving naturally. The Western approach is to diagnose using a process of elimination and a series of tests. It is an excellent way to identify problems such as blocked fallopian tubes.

THE FIRST ZHAI CLINIC BABY

PROBLEM:	**inability to conceive for 7 years**
METHODS TRIED:	**5 IVF cycles**
INVESTIGATION:	**laparoscopy, hormone tests, ultrasound scan and semen analysis**
MENSTRUAL CYCLE:	**regular**

SYMPTOMS:	**significant premenstrual tension**
HUSBAND:	**slightly low sperm count**
TCM OBJECTIVE:	**to clear Liver stagnation**
LENGTH OF TREATMENT:	**4 months**
OUTCOME:	**natural conception; a healthy baby**

I will always remember my very first patient (I will call her May). She was referred to me by a colleague, Dr Luo, who was renowned for her skills in treating dermatological complaints. A woman in her late 30s had approached her to ask whether TCM can help infertility. Dr Luo was so busy she was unable to see her so she recommended me.

In May's case there were no particular hormonal issues, she had regular periods and although her husband's sperm count was slightly low, her ovarian reserve was average. Her infertility really was unexplained. However, she reported having a lot of premenstrual tension (PMT), so we focused on helping her to balance her body health and to clear the Liver stagnation. If the Liver is not working, the whole system will cease to function properly.

After just four months, May became pregnant. I was almost as astonished as she was. The result led me to undertake some research into fertility treatments in Western countries – what options are available for infertile couples and how successful they are. I wanted to learn the best method for treating infertility, how far research had developed into the causes and what Western medicine could and couldn't do. My first patient set me on my path to become an infertility specialist in Britain. That was in 1995–6. Since then, I have shared the joy of over 1,000 babies being born using Zhai TCM treatments.

In contrast, when I first take on a patient, I try to understand why the body's metabolism isn't working properly and I use TCM to determine a treatment plan. My main tools for diagnosis are an extensive lifestyle questionnaire (see pages 251–258), tongue and pulse diagnosis (see pages 32–33), and the results of the Western-style tests and analyses that have been performed.

Before I explain how I use my treatment methods, I'd like to look at the causes of the most common fertility problems.

In Western medicine the causes of infertility tend to be classed in three categories:

- Problems with the ovaries (see pages 89–92)
- Problems with the fallopian tubes (see pages 93–94)
- Male infertility problems (see pages 98–101)

As many as 30 per cent of fertility problems have multiple causes and some are termed 'unexplained', when doctors can't pin down exactly what is wrong.

Problems with the ovaries

There are many problems associated with the ovaries that can cause infertility; these are some of the most common.

The female reproductive system

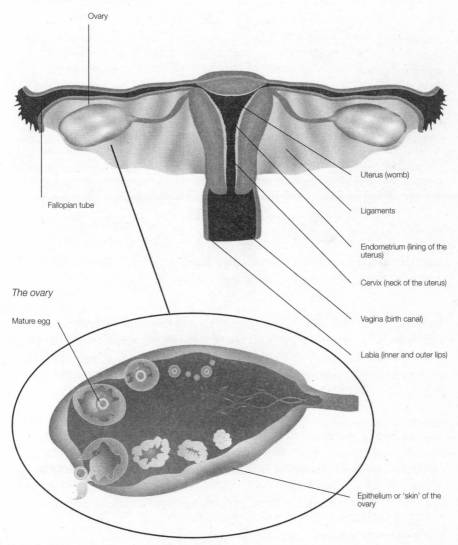

Ovary

Fallopian tube

Uterus (womb)

Ligaments

Endometrium (lining of the uterus)

Cervix (neck of the uterus)

Vagina (birth canal)

Labia (inner and outer lips)

The ovary

Mature egg

Epithelium or 'skin' of the ovary

AGE

We all know that a woman's age affects her fertility levels and there is a well-documented decline in the female body's ability to form an egg cell as it ages. Generally speaking, there is a ten-year period called the peri-menopause, between the ages of 35 and 45, during which a woman's egg quality and egg production are in decline.

Not only does the number of eggs decline with a woman's age, but so too does their quality. So even if an IVF cycle in a fertility clinic appears to produce a clutch of eggs, it may be that they are immature or fragmented, or the sperm swim away from the egg because the egg cell is too hard for the sperm to penetrate.

PREMATURE OVARIAN FAILURE (POF)

Premature ovarian failure is diagnosed when a woman under the age of 40 has stopped having periods for four months or more and blood tests reveal her follicle stimulating hormone (FSH) levels are in the menopausal range. POF may also result if the woman's ovaries malfunction, causing follicle production to degenerate at a faster rate than normal.

There can be many reasons, single or multiple, for POF and it is often impossible to pinpoint the cause. It may run in families so it's useful to know the age that your mother went through the menopause, because you may have a genetic predisposition.

POF has also been associated with other genetic defects, infections such as mumps or could be the result of medical treatments such as radiotherapy and chemotherapy. The body's own immune system may well play a part and doctors might look for evidence of this, as well as illnesses such as Addison's disease (a condition of the andrenal glands) or thyroid problems.

In some rare cases the body can restart its ovarian function naturally, especially if it is recovering from a lot of stress or dramatic weight loss.

HYPERPROLACTINEMIA

High levels of the hormone prolactin in the blood stream can prevent the ovaries from releasing eggs. During pregnancy and while a woman is breastfeeding, prolactin is produced by the pituitary gland to prepare the breasts for lactation. That's why women are often told they won't get pregnant again while they are breastfeeding, although this is not a reliable method of contraception.

But high levels of prolactin can also be an indication of problems such as a pituitary tumour, or can be induced by taking tranquillizers or certain drugs to treat high blood pressure. It is still possible for ovulation to occur if the level of prolactin is not too high, but even a slightly raised level can interfere with the hormone function of the corpus luteum, causing insufficient progesterone to support the next stage of successful fertilization.

HYPOTHALAMIC AMENORRHEA

The hypothalamus is a part of the brain that helps control the secretion of hormones. Hypothalamic amenorrhea occurs when the hypothalamus fails to send the pituitary gland the right messages necessary to stimulate ovulation.

Although in many patients the underlying cause of this condition is not known, certain things can contribute to it, including weight loss, extreme exercise, stress and the use of narcotic drugs.

LUTEAL PHASE DEFECT

Luteal phase defect (LPD) occurs when the luteal phase of the cycle is too short. It can be difficult to diagnose but it's an indication that the corpus luteum isn't secreting sufficient progesterone, the hormone essential for successful implantation and early maintenance of a pregnancy.

Although it isn't considered a common cause of infertility it may be a significant factor in certain patients, for example women who experience repeated miscarriages.

Progesterone deficiency can be the result of too little being produced, or because production is not maintained over a long enough period of time. It is seen more often at the beginning or end of a woman's reproductive life and has been linked to excessive exercise, extreme weight and hyperandrogenism (an excessive production of the hormones, androgens). It is often treated by the administration of high levels of human chorionic gonadotropin (HCG) at the ovulation stage, or during IVF.

POLYCYSTIC OVARY SYNDROME (PCOS)

PCOS is one of the most common causes of infertility and is due to a hormonal imbalance. It can have a strong genetic link, often running through several generations of a family, especially if there is also a history of diabetes and high cholesterol in the family.

Polycystic ovaries become covered in small cysts. These are egg-containing follicles that haven't matured sufficiently to produce a viable egg. Although the cysts themselves are harmless, it's a sign that the hormones aren't working well enough to trigger ovulation, or do so only occasionally.

Why the hormone imbalance occurs isn't exactly understood but it can have other consequences. It can lead to raised levels of luteinizing hormone and male hormones such as testosterone, and reduced levels of follicle stimulating hormone and progesterone. The raise in testosterone levels can cause some women with polycystic ovaries to have excess body hair and skin problems such as acne.

PCOS is also linked to insulin resistance. Insulin is the hormone that regulates the breakdown of sugar in the body. As the body becomes resistant to insulin, the pancreas has to produce more of it. Raised insulin levels trigger the production of more testosterone, which interferes with ovulation. Raised insulin also causes the body to store more fat (particularly around the middle), and fat stores trigger the body to release more insulin in a vicious circle.

Not everyone with polycystic ovaries will have the hormone imbalance that indicates Polycystic Ovary Syndrome. In fact it is quite common for women to have cysts in their ovaries.

THYROID FUNCTION

In some cases, an over- or underactive thyroid may cause infertility. The thyroid secretes the hormones thyroxine and triiodothyronine, which regulate the body's metabolism, heart rate and temperature.

An overactive thyroid gland (hyperthyroidism) increases the body's metabolism, which has been linked to an increased chance of miscarriage, possibly because the metabolic rate speeds up the breakdown of progesterone, so the pregnancy won't thrive.

An underactive thyroid gland (hypothyroidism) does the opposite, slowing down the metabolism. In severe cases this can cause ovarian failure.

The production of thyroxine can also be affected by treatments for thyroid cancer, too little iodine in the diet, viral illnesses, drug reactions and abnormalities of the pituitary gland.

Autoimmune thyroiditis may also be a cause of premature ovarian failure (the loss of ovarian function before the age of 40) (see page 90).

Case study

Chloe, aged 38

PROBLEM:	**severe PCOS**
METHODS TRIED:	**2 IUI cycles, 3 ICSI cycles**
TCM OBJECTIVE:	**to regulate the menstrual cycle**
LENGTH OF TREATMENT:	**2 years**
OUTCOME:	**natural conception; 2 children in the long term**

Chloe had been diagnosed with severe PCOS at quite a young age. She hadn't met her husband until she was 30, so was feeling that she'd left it too late to become pregnant. She was 38 when she came to the clinic, following two IUI cycles and three failed ICSI cycles. Her periods occurred only about every nine months.

TCM assessment and treatment plan

Chloe was overweight, her tongue was pale and sticky and her pulse was weak and slippery. Her consultant was very supportive of her trying TCM to improve her cycle, especially as she had insulin resistance and was taking Metformin (a diabetes inhibitor). Her husband's sperm count was in the normal range and he was very calm and confident that they would have a baby, however long it took.

I started treatment with herbal tea and acupuncture. Chloe's first cycle was 77 days; the next reduced to 72. Over the next six to seven cycles, the cycle length reduced by about five days each time. Eventually she reached a point where she had two cycles of 35 days, and she was ready to try again with assisted fertility treatment. However, at that point she conceived naturally. She later went on to have a second baby after using Metformin to treat her insulin resistance.

Problems with the fallopian tubes

Problems associated with the fallopian tubes and surrounding tissue are very common causes of infertility, and they can often be successfully treated by surgery or assisted conception treatments provided the problem is not associated with ovarian malfunction.

BLOCKAGE IN THE TUBES

The fallopian tubes are the passageways through which the sperm travel to the eggs for fertilization, and the eggs travel from the ovaries to the womb. Normally, the ovaries each release a single egg on alternate months. Although they look thin and delicate, the fallopian tubes are actually strong and have layers of muscle which help propel the egg on its journey.

A blockage in the fallopian tubes obviously makes the physical act of fertilization difficult if not impossible. There are many causes of tubal blockage, but also many successful ways of treating it. IVF was developed specifically to bypass any blockages in the fallopian tubes; this is one of the conditions most successfully treated by assisted conception.

Scarring and adhesions on the fallopian tubes can also cause problems with fertility. These can be caused by inflammation due to infection, especially if left untreated. This is why it is so important to have treatment for any sexually transmitted disease such as chlamydia or gonorrhoea as soon as they are diagnosed. Even a yeast infection can cause damage if left untreated.

Some studies also reveal that fertility problems can occur even if just one fallopian tube is blocked. If the blockage is at the end of the tube next to the ovary (the fimbrial end), there is a possibility that fluid will build up inside the tube and have no means to drain away (a condition known as hydrosalpinx). Fluid could flood into the uterus, washing away any fertilized eggs that have implanted there naturally or through IVF.

ENDOMETRIOSIS

The womb is lined with endometrial cells which are sensitive to changes in oestrogen and progesterone levels. The cells grow during the menstrual cycle, then are shed as a monthly 'period' bleed if no fertilized egg implants in the womb. In some women, endometrial-like cells grow outside the womb, most commonly around the fallopian tubes and ovaries but they can also be present in the abdomen, affecting the vagina, bowel and bladder.

These cells behave in a similar way to those inside the womb, growing and breaking down each month. But unlike those in the womb, they cannot be shed outside the body. They cause an internal inflammatory reaction which, in turn, causes the painful, heavy periods, abdominal pain and bleeding between periods that sufferers of endometriosis will recognise only too well.

In Western medicine, there is not much discussion about the causes of endometriosis although it is considered likely to stem from genetic, hormonal and immunity factors. There's no cure as such, but the problems can be alleviated by laser treatment.

The problem for women with endometriosis who want to conceive is that as well as damaging the tubes, the endometrial-like cells can produce chemicals which attack the sperm and prevent the egg from being fertilized. Once pregnant, however, women with endometriosis should not find that the condition puts the pregnancy at risk.

The TCM view of endometriosis does not relate to genetic factors; it is an obstruction caused by Blood stasis that allows the deposit to grow and stay in the abdominal environment. The abdominal environment needs to be cleared in order to get the Blood flow moving and rebuild the reproductive system.

Other causes of female infertility

Most female infertility problems are associated with the ovaries and fallopian tubes, but there are other possible problems too.

PROBLEMS IN THE WOMB

Fibroids or polyps growing inside the uterus (womb) can be a physical barrier to a successful pregnancy and should be easy to detect using modern scanning devices. Although large fibroids may limit the size of the cavity area in which an egg can implant, experts are not yet sure whether smaller fibroids interfere with fertility, although it's possible that polyps could interfere with the development of the endometrial lining.

CERVICAL PROBLEMS

Just as hormonal changes control what is happening in the ovaries and uterus, they also assist the sperm's journey towards the egg by providing a healthy environment in the cervix. If the mucus in the cervix is thick, sticky or too acid when the sperm are trying to pass through, it makes their journey to the womb and up to a waiting egg much more difficult.

Cervical or vaginal infections can cause a discharge which can also hamper fertility, and in some cases previous surgery or scarring to the cervix can cause problems.

INFLAMMATION OF THE PELVIC ORGANS

Pelvic Inflammatory Disease (PID) is an infection of the reproductive organs such as the uterus, fallopian tubes and ovaries. It's usually caused by a bacterial infection which may have started in the vagina or cervix but has now spread further. The cause of the infection is often a sexually transmitted disease, such as chlamydia, but as the disease may produce no symptoms many women leave it untreated for many years. If the infection spreads to the reproductive organs, it can develop into a number of conditions, all of which affect fertility.

Such an infection can cause inflammation of the endometrium and womb (endometriosis); inflammation and infection of the fallopian tubes (salpingitis); and inflammation of the ovaries and tissue surrounding the womb. It can also cause abscesses on the ovaries and fallopian tubes or even pelvic peritonitis.

Antibiotics can quickly clear PID if it is caught early. If left untreated or not properly healed, it may contribute towards ectopic pregnancy, in which the foetus develops outside the womb.

NATURAL KILLER CELLS

Natural killer (NK) cells are a type of lymphocyte (white blood cell) that form part of the body's immune system. The role of the immune system is to fight any 'foreign' cells that it doesn't recognize, which may be threatening the body. There are cells in the womb lining that are similar to NK cells, so they are known as uterine NK cells. Their role seems to be to help the placenta connect to the mother's blood vessels.

There is a theory being currently investigated that if women repeatedly suffer from miscarriage, uterine NK cells may be playing a part in rejecting the pregnancy. The uterine NK cells may see the developing foetus (which has a different genetic make-up to its mother) as a threat to the body and act to prevent its development. The assumption is that in a healthy pregnancy the immune response is suppressed to allow the foetus to develop without harm. However, the latest discussion at the Human Fertilization and Embryology Authority (HDEA) suggests there is no convincing evidence to support this. I am keeping an open mind, but am currently very cautious about accepting the theory. It would be more convincing and helpful if there had also been studies on healthy pregnant women with no history of miscarriage, to see whether natural killer cells are found in their blood and uterus during pregnancy.

NK cell tests and treatments are very new and are not licensed for use in reproductive medicine. The clinical trials to date have involved very small numbers of women. However, there are a number of doctors who are suggesting that it is possible to use a blood test to assess high levels of NK cells and that drugs can then be used to suppress them. I have seen many patients who have been on these treatments for more than a year or two. Although the NK cells may have been suppressed, no pregnancy has been achieved. Any sensible fertility doctor should acknowledge that 98–99 per cent of pregnancies rely on a healthy egg and sperm forming a healthy embryo and achieving a healthy pregnancy. If this has not been achieved, it is hard to believe a pregnancy is even possible.

If you have an interest in the subject, the HFEA website (www.hfea.gov.uk) is a useful source of information.

Case study

Kitty, aged 37/George, aged 45

PROBLEMS:	**high NK cell count/severely low sperm count**
METHODS TRIED:	**3 ICSI cycles, FET**
TCM OBJECTIVE:	**to improve the health of the uterus/to clear Damp and Heat in the lower abdomen**
LENGTH OF TREATMENT:	**4 months**
OUTCOME:	**natural conception**

Kitty was 37 and George was 45 years old when they came to visit us. Due to George's severely low sperm count, low sperm motility and a high percentage of sperm with abnormal form, the couple had been advised that their only chance of conceiving would be via ICSI. They had conceived successfully following their first ICSI cycle and had a three-year-old son. When they decided to try for a second child, they had three further ICSI cycles and one frozen embryo transfer but no pregnancy was achieved. The couple hoped that TCM support might help them to maximize their chances of success if they began another ICSI cycle.

TCM assessment and treatment plan

Kitty had an excellent hormone profile, with normal levels of FSH, LH, oestradiol, prolactin, Anti-Mullerian hormone and inhibin B. However, she had a raised level of natural killer (NK) cells. Her periods were regular but very painful, which indicated to us at the clinic that a course of treatment to remove Blood stasis would be beneficial, to help implantation to some degree. I could also see that her husband would benefit from treatment.

I discussed with the couple whether they would like to try TCM for three months to benefit Kitty's blood flow and to improve George's semen quality and quantity before attempting another cycle of ICSI.

George was slightly overweight and drank more than 15 units of alcohol per week. His bowel movements were loose and frequent; he slept a lot and tired easily. He had a white, thick, rough tongue that was typical of Damp and Heat symptoms, which sink to the lower abdomen causing obstruction. Because of this, his digestive system worked under pressure. Unhealthy fluids stayed in the lower part of his body for a long time, restricting the levels of oxygen and nutrition necessary for healthy sperm production – which was contributing to the low sperm count, low motility and high levels of abnormal sperm.

To ease his digestive system, I asked George to stop drinking alcohol completely and to avoid eating greasy, spicy foods, or having cold or chilled drinks. Following three weeks of herbal medication, George reported that his stools were not as loose and his bowel movements were less frequent. He was less sleepy and less fatigued. After eight weeks of herbal medication, George reported that he still had three bowel movements per day but they were not loose like before. He felt well and was no longer constantly fatigued.

We planned for the couple to complete TCM treatment at least three months before starting their next ICSI cycle. However, on completion of three months of TCM treatment and just before she was due to start the ICSI cycle the following month, Kitty discovered that she had conceived naturally. Interestingly, this time there was no need for an anti-NK cell drug as a blood test showed her NK cell level to be normal. I continued to treat Kitty until the thirteenth week of her pregnancy.

Male infertility problems

Abnormal sperm is the most common cause of infertility in men, so semen analysis remains the primary screening test (see pages 83–85).

The male reproductive system

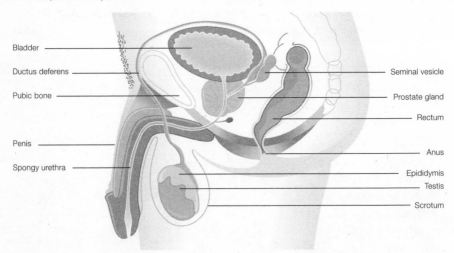

Bladder
Ductus deferens
Pubic bone
Penis
Spongy urethra

Seminal vesicle
Prostate gland
Rectum
Anus
Epididymis
Testis
Scrotum

SPERM QUANTITY

The sperm count (sperm concentration) should be at least 15 million per millilitre (ml) of semen (the liquid in which sperm is carried) or 39 million per sample. Various factors may cause a decreased sperm count, including hormone imbalances, genetic factors, infections, age, heat exposure, stress and obesity, as well as lifestyle factors.

An absence of sperm in the semen (a condition known as azoospermia) can be due to a blockage in one of the tubes that make up the reproductive system, which may have been caused by an infection or surgery. It could also be caused by testicular failure, something a further male infertility test or testicular biopsy may be able to confirm.

SPERM QUALITY

The number of sperm will obviously have an effect on fertility, but so will the quality. Decreased sperm motility makes it harder for the sperm to swim to the egg. At least 40 per cent of the sperm should be motile. Thirty-two per cent should be swimming progressively forward towards the egg (see box, below).

Abnormal-shaped sperm may be less able to move properly, making it harder for them to fertilize an egg. Causes of poor structure include genetic predisposition, heat damage, stress, lifestyle factors, anabolic steroids and environmental toxins.

Environmental pollutants such as dioxins, pesticides such as DDT, or solvents used in paints, can act like oestrogens or anti-androgens and have been shown to have a harmful effect on sperm. Although many have been withdrawn from sale there is still a concern that certain pesticides and chemicals are still contaminating the food chain and exposing men to these substances.

The methods used to assess the quality of sperm differ between testing laboratories and opinion about the value of these tests is divided.

SPERM TEST RESULTS

The results of a healthy sperm test will fall within the range of figures below.

Volume of semen	greater than 1.5 ml
Total number of sperm	39 million per sample
Concentration of sperm	15 million per ml
Total sperm motility	40%
Progressive sperm motility	32%
Live spermatozoa	58%
Normal (healthy) sperm	4%

Adapted from the World Health Organization's *Manual for Semen Analysis*, 2010)

PROBLEMS WITH THE TESTICLES

Sperm is produced and stored in the testicles and if these are damaged it may affect the quality of the semen. Damage to the testicles can be the result of:

- **Infection of the testicles**

- **Testicular surgery or injury**

- **Congenital defect**

- **Undescended testicles** When one or both testicles have not descended into the scrotum but remain inside the abdomen or the inguinal canal. The reason the testicles don't descend remains unclear, though a number of risk factors have been identified and include genetic factors, such as being born prematurely, a low birth weight, maternal diabetes and smoking or alcohol consumption by the mother during pregnancy.

- **Testicular lumps and swelling** This may be due to a cyst in the epididymis (the fine tube through which the sperm leave the testicles); inflammation of the scrotum, caused by injury, infection, or radiotherapy; testicular torsion (when the testicle rotates within its sac, cutting off its own blood supply), which requires immediate medical intervention; or varicoceles, a mass of varicose veins supplying the testicles, which do not circulate blood efficiently. This leads to an accumulation of blood, which causes swelling.

- **Testicular cancer** The causes are unknown, but risk factors that have been identified include: family history, being born with undescended testicles, age and smoking.

STERILIZATION
A vasectomy may be reversed, but reversals may not always be successful.

EJACULATION DISORDERS
Premature ejaculation (where ejaculation occurs too quickly) or retrograde ejaculation (where semen is ejaculated into the bladder) can make it difficult for men to ejaculate semen into the vagina and can obviously affect fertility. There may be an underlying medical cause for these conditions, so it is wise to check this with your family doctor.

HYPOGONADISM
Hypogonadism is another possible cause of infertility. It is defined as an abnormally low level of testosterone, the hormone involved in making sperm. Causes include a tumour or Kallmann's syndrome (a rare disorder which is caused by a faulty gene).

MEDICINES AND DRUGS
Some medicines can have side effects that lead to infertility problems, such as the anti-inflammatory medicine Sulfasalazine, anabolic steroids and chemotherapy.

ALCOHOL

Alcohol abuse has been shown to damage the quality of sperm.

TREATING MALE INFERTILITY

There is growing evidence that TCM can significantly improve sperm quantity and quality and I shall deal with this in a later chapter. So, before turning to expensive and intrusive methods of treatment, I advise men to at least try TCM because the results can be fast, impressive and painless (although some Chinese herbal tea concoctions aren't to everyone's taste). It is vital, however, to ensure that the woman's fertile health is at its peak at the same time, so I recommend both the man and the woman are treated.

Chapter 6

THE TCM APPROACH TO INFERTILITY

TCM looks at the wider picture of human health, including emotional and mental balance, to make a diagnosis. It also takes into consideration what the patient has inherited from his or her parents (known in TCM as *jing*, see page 23), as this can have a bearing on fertility levels.

INTERNAL CAUSES OF INFERTILITY BEFORE BIRTH

- **Weak constitution** A person is born with a certain constitution, which is inherited from the parents and contributes to his or her health and development as an embryo in the mother's womb. For example, some women undergo premature menopause in their late 20s, and others can have a baby at the age of 50. Likewise, some men can father a child but by the age of 40 their sperm is drastically reduced, while others become fathers at the age of 70. This difference may be down to a difference in constitution.

Although the individual's inherited constitution, by and large, cannot be changed, it can be improved within certain limits by having a healthy and balanced lifestyle, and practising breathing exercises to regenerate one's health.

INTERNAL CAUSES OF INFERTILITY AFTER BIRTH

- **Emotions** As we have seen, in TCM, there are Seven Emotions: Joy, Anger, Anxiety, Pensiveness, Sorrow, Fear and Fright (see pages 30–31). Under normal circumstances, emotions should not cause health problems, but if an emotion is sudden, intense or persistent over a long period it can cause dysfunction in the internal organs, result in disharmony of *yin* and *yang*, *qi* and Blood, and cause diseases.

It is understood in TCM that extreme emotional changes can bring about different influences on the internal organs. There is an accepted saying in TCM, that *'Anger injures the Liver, Joy injures the Heart, Pensiveness injures the Spleen, Sorrow injures the Lung, Fear injures the Kidney.'*

Some symptoms commonly caused by emotions are insomnia or disturbed sleep, palpitations, depression, irritable bowel syndrome, a sensation of obstruction in the throat and menstrual irregularities.

- **Excessive activity** Excessive mental and physical activity includes working too hard, over-exercising and too much sexual activity.

Normal physical labour is beneficial to the smooth and healthy running of the human body and can increase physical strength and prevent illness. Excessive activity can overwork and weaken the body's constitution and indirectly causes Kidney deficiency.

- **Poor diet** Irregular intake of food or an improper amount of certain foods, including too much alcohol, spicy food, coffee, tobacco and cold drinks and foods, will exceed the digestive ability of the human body and could weaken or damage the organs, in particular the Spleen and Stomach. If the food cannot be broken down, transported and transformed, it can lead to symptoms of Spleen *qi* deficiency and malnutrition of the body.

EXTERNAL CAUSES

- **Climatic factors** In normal circumstances, the weather will have no effect on the human body, as the body can adjust itself to changing conditions and protect itself against external disease-causing factors. However, when the balance between the body and the environment breaks down, the weather can become a cause of disease, either because the weather is unseasonably excessive or because the body is weak, or relatively weaker than the climatic changes (see pages 30–31).

An excessive climatic change that brings disease can completely change the body's nature, leading to disharmony and causing malfunction in the reproductive organs.

OTHER CAUSES

- **Trauma** Having an ovarian cyst, tumour or fibroid removed, an operation for undescended testicles, varicocele or vasectomy – or indeed any operation – can cause trauma to the body and impair the working of the ovaries and testicles, especially if the appropriate aftercare is not taken.

- **Chemical** Chemotherapy and radiotherapy disrupt the reproductive organs. Over the last 15 years, many articles have also reported that contaminated water, plastic containers, GM products and plastic bags that contain oestrogen may have a chemical effect on fertility.

- **Infection** Genital tract infections and sexually transmitted diseases, such as chlamydia, and Pelvic Inflammatory Disease (PID) can cause abnormalities in the abdominal environment, such as blocked fallopian tubes, the development of adhesions and sperm production problems.

Infertility patterns in women

Although the Western classifications of infertility described earlier do not translate directly into TCM equivalents, their symptoms are easily analysed and categorized to fit a TCM diagnostic pattern. In TCM, infertility is generally categorized into excess or deficient patterns (see page 22), and it is important when diagnosing infertility to differentiate clearly between the two. However, deficient and excess patterns often coexist so the diagnosis will look at the relationship between the two patterns.

EXCESS PATTERNS

Excess patterns obstruct the organs of the abdomen, particularly the woman's ovaries and womb, the Conception and Penetrating Vessels (see pages 51–52), preventing qi, Blood and essence circulating, and slowing down the transformation of food into energy so that egg quality is affected and fertilization cannot occur.

Excess patterns could obstruct the womb, causing a blockage, so that implantation cannot occur. TCM describes this as Blood stagnation, and it varies in degree, from mild (the Blood is retarded) through to severe (complete Blood stasis), with various complications.

Dampness in lower *jiao* (abdomen)

Dampness in the abdomen may be due to extreme weather conditions, such as rain or humidity, or overconsumption of greasy, cold or damp foods, such as dairy products, sugar, fatty foods, alcohol, iced drinks or cold drinks straight from the fridge. These can cause the Stomach and Spleen to either overwork or work too slowly, resulting in the body retaining too much fluid and becoming Damp.

Dampness impairs the Spleen's ability to transform and transport food and drink (the lining of stomach becomes inflamed) and so leads to the production of internal Dampness and eventually the formation of Phlegm. Dampness accumulates and due to its heavy, sinking tendency it flows downwards, collecting in the abdomen and blocking healthy Blood circulation in the reproductive system. This sometimes leads to a larger than normal ovary (in the case of polycystic ovaries or PCOS), or a 'Damp uterus' with impaired function, so fertilization is prevented or implantation is difficult.

Symptoms: Dampness is often associated with deficient Spleen qi and is commonly seen in patients who present with polycystic ovaries or PCOS, or restricted sperm production. Patients often complain of feeling sleepy, sleep heavily or need long hours of sleep and produce loose stools. Dampness will also show itself in a prolonged and irregular menstrual cycle, tiredness, infertility that has persisted for a long time already, abundant yellow vaginal discharge in women, a swollen tongue or a tongue with teeth marks, a pale and sticky tongue and a weak and slippery pulse.

Over time, Dampness frequently combines with Heat, giving rise to Damp-Heat, or Phlegm-Heat, which causes further obstruction and can form endometriosis and ovarian cysts.

Liver *Qi* stagnation

Emotion is the most common cause of *qi* stagnation, particularly anxiety, stress and anger. In TCM, the Liver is considered to have the same functions and roles as those attributed to it in Western medicine. The Liver's primary function is to store Blood and regulate the amount of Blood that various parts of the body receive. It also encourages a smooth and uninterrupted flow of *qi* to help the Blood circulate throughout the body.

The Liver Meridian (see page 50) starts at the big toe, goes up the inside of the leg to the pubic region, encircles the genitals, then enters the lower abdomen, where it connects with the stomach, gall bladder and liver. Liver *qi* stagnation inhibits the flow of Liver *qi*. It has a great influence over menstrual cycles in women and also plays a very important part in assisting successful ovulation and conception.

Other causes that can contribute to *qi* stagnation are stagnant food due to overeating, Blood stasis due to trauma, long-term Blood deficiency and Dampness, as these may all impede the free flow of *qi*.

Symptoms: *Qi* stagnation is commonly seen in patients who have been diagnosed with immunological infertility (a controversial diagnosis that supports the idea that natural killer (NK) cells may play a part in causing miscarriage. See page 96.) Symptoms include severe premenstrual tension, mood swings or depression, elevated prolactin or headaches before periods, extreme breast tenderness and a bloated stomach. They may display a purple tongue and a wiry or choppy pulse.

Blood stasis

Blood stasis obstructs the human body. When it obstructs the abdomen, healthy Blood flow is restricted, affecting the normal function of the ovaries and womb. This stagnation or blockage will also prevent an egg or sperm from entering the womb and menstrual blood from draining out freely.

Blood stasis in the lower abdomen is common in women as the womb is said to store Blood. It may be caused by a trauma such as lack of appropriate care after abdominal surgery, Blood deficiency, abortion, intercourse during menstruation, incomplete discharge of menstrual blood and residual blood after giving birth. Prolonged *qi* stagnation is a major cause of Blood stasis, and emotional and mental factors can play an important role in this.

Cold invasion may also be a cause of Blood stasis, as Cold congeals Blood, just as Cold congeals water in nature. So wearing inadequate clothing in cold climates or consuming too many cold or raw foods can be a problem. A further cause of Blood stasis in TCM is Blood Heat as Heat consumes body fluids and may cause the Blood to thicken and clot. The most frequent causes of Blood Heat are prolonged Liver *qi* stagnation transforming into Fire, excessive consumption of hot, spicy foods and a deficiency of *yin*, leading to deficient Heat (Heat created by a deficiency).

Symptoms: Blood stasis and *qi* stagnation can be complicated by Phlegm-Damp, a combination that is found in patients with endometriosis, blockage of the fallopian tubes, scarring of organ tissue, ovarian cysts and fibroids in the womb (uterine myomas). The combination of Damp-Heat (see page 126) or Heat toxins with Blood stasis is found in patients with infections in the cervix, vagina or fallopian tubes. Patients with Blood stasis often complain of cold limbs, painful menstrual cycles or abdominal pain after ovulation and during the second half of the menstrual cycle.

Blood Heat

Heat consumes body fluids and so the Blood, in effect, thickens and may start to clot. It is usually due to Liver Heat or Liver Fire, which is passed to the Blood, making it 'hot'. The most typical cause of this excess pattern is Liver *qi* stagnation. As explained above, *qi* is naturally warm so if it builds up excessively, as it does with *qi* stagnation, it easily turns into disease-producing Heat or Fire. Also, the overconsumption of meat, cheese, hot and spicy foods and alcohol can provoke the development of Heat from *qi* stagnation.

On the other hand, Blood Heat may also cause excessive bleeding and threaten miscarriage. In some cases Blood Heat is caused by the constitution with which a person was born.

Symptoms: Blood Heat is commonly seen in women with a short menstrual cycle, early ovulation and heavy menstrual blood loss. It is also commonly seen in women whose follicles grow too fast during an IVF cycle, when they may only have had a few days of follicle stimulating hormone injections, or in women who ovulate before egg collection can take place.

Cold

External Cold can directly affect a woman's womb, particularly during puberty, menstruation and after giving birth. Once Cold invades the body it turns into internal Cold. If this Cold is not dispersed quickly it will consume the body's *yang*, so turning the body from an excess Cold pattern into a deficient *yang* type. Too many raw, cold and iced foods and drinks may also lead to Cold in the womb by chilling the Fire of digestion.

Symptoms: A Cold womb is commonly seen in women with a prolonged menstrual cycle and late ovulation who respond slowly to drugs during an IVF cycle – even though there are many small follicles present; or in those who experience repeated miscarriage and implantation failure.

DEFICIENT TYPES

Deficiencies (see below) may reduce fertility. To maximize your chances of getting pregnant you should have strong Kidney *jing* and a good balance between Kidney *yin* and Kidney *yang*, Blood and *qi*, and be free from any obstruction in the body, particularly the abdomen.

Jing is sometimes referred to as the 'reproductive essence' and is said to be inherited from one's parents (see page 23). In Western medicine, the nearest equivalent is probably 'constitution', but as ever this is a loose translation. The important thing is that, in addition to defining your 'constitution', *jing* affects your ability to have children, so having a plentiful supply of this particular energy is vital.

Because *jing* is inherited, you may find that if your parents were in poor health, they smoke, drank or took drugs, your constitution may be at risk and have a low level of *jing*. This doesn't mean that you are genetically disposed to be infertile or ill, but it's an indication of what sort of measures you might want to take to achieve better health. And, of course, the healthier you are as a potential parent the better the *jing* you will pass on to your children. As in most areas of fertility, *jing* declines with age.

Kidney deficiency

In TCM, conception is seen as a blending of the energies of the woman and the man to form what the Chinese call 'pre-heaven essence' or the 'seed' of the newly conceived baby. This essence forms the healthy egg, nourishes the developing baby during pregnancy and determines the hereditary constitution, strength and vitality of the child. Although the amount and quality of this form of essence is fixed at birth, it can be restored and enhanced through a lifestyle with a good balance of work and rest, through breathing exercises and a balanced diet. This essence forms the basis for growth, development, reproductive function and fertility. It is referred to as the Kidney essence in Chinese medicine as it is stored in the Kidney, but due to its fluid nature it also circulates throughout the meridians in the body, particularly through the Extraordinary Vessels (see pages 51–52).

The weakness may be due to:

- A constitutional *jing* weakness if the parents' constitution was not good and/or the parents' health was not good at the time of conception.
- A natural decline of essence as a result of ageing.
- Excessive sexual activity at an early age (before and during puberty), which seriously depletes Kidney essence and damages the Conception and Penetrating Vessels (see pages 51–52). This can cause infertility later in life.

Kidney essence is closely related to Kidney *yin* and Kidney *yang*, the fundamental balancing system for the whole body. The *yin* and the *yang* aspects of the essence need to be in perfect balance for fertilization to occur. The *yin* essence provides the basis for conception by producing the egg, while the *yang* has a warming and fertilizing role and is essential for the transformation of the egg into a foetus.

Symptoms: If the Kidney essence is weak, a young woman may start her periods late and fail to ovulate or have irregular ovulation due to poorly functioning ovaries.

Kidney *yin* deficiency

Because *yin* is naturally fluid-like (Blood is an aspect of *yin*), it is associated with the nourishing and moistening body functions. *Yin* is also closely allied to essence (see page 107).

Kidney *yin* forms the basis for menstrual blood and menstrual function and can be related to the ovum (egg) and the corpus luteum. If Kidney *yin* is deficient, the womb and related meridians will lack the necessary nourishment to nurture the egg. The relevant meridians are the Conception and Penetrating Vessels, which are *yin* in nature (see pages 51–52).

A deficiency of Kidney *yin* may be caused by a constitutional tendency, but it also naturally declines with age. However, *yin* may be consumed more rapidly by some lifestyle factors, including overwork, a poor diet, inadequate sleep and exercise, and chronic disease. So, working long hours without adequate rest and with an irregular diet over a long period of time is a common cause for the consumption of Kidney *yin* in today's society.

Due to the close relationship between Blood and *yin*, loss of large quantities of blood, for example through heavy periods or surgery, also depletes *yin*. And inadequate protein in the diet can cause Blood depletion, which explains why a balanced diet is so important in fertility treatment.

Symptoms: Patients with Kidney *yin* deficiency tend to have long-term infertility. When it is associated with *qi* stagnation it will cause problems with ovulation, such as a failure to ovulate, elevated FSH and poor response to the follicle stimulating drugs during IVF. Symptoms of *yin* deficiency also include feelings of Heat, hot cheeks, night sweating, dry mucous membranes (in the nose, eyes and mouth), a weak lower back and delayed, scanty and light-coloured menstruation. Patients may also have a red tongue and a rapid or fine pulse.

Kidney *yang* deficiency

Yang balances *yin* and in contrast to *yin* is active and warming, with *qi* being an aspect of *yang*. *Yang* aids ovulation and the free movement of the egg. In particular, Kidney *yang* or Kidney Fire provides the 'spark' for essence to fertilize and nourish the egg, while also warming the womb and the entire body. *Yang* provides the force of transformation that assists fertilization, that is the maturation of follicles, the release of the egg and the maturation of the corpus luteum.

Excessive physical work and strenuous exercise, especially at puberty when the womb is in a vulnerable state, weakens *yang* and Kidney and Spleen *yang* in particular. Kidney Fire or Kidney *yang* can also be weakened or exhausted by genital weakness, chronic illness, fatigue and exhaustion and the ageing process.

Symptoms: Kidney *yang* deficiency is commonly seen in patients with a history of repeated miscarriage and lack of monthly periods. Patients often complain of feeling cold, having chills in the four limbs, urgent stools, frequent or night urination, delayed menstruation and low libido. They will show a pale and wet tongue, and deep and slow pulse.

Blood deficiency

According to TCM, Blood is produced by the Spleen from the food we eat and transformed into menstrual blood and breast milk in women. So every case of Blood deficiency can also be attributed to Spleen deficiency. In turn, the Liver's function in storing and regulating the volume of Blood is fundamental in gynaecology as this regulates menstruation and the amount of Blood stored in the womb, and the Conception and Penetrating Vessels (see pages 51–52).

Blood and essence (see page 107) influence one another, as essence can be transformed into Blood while Blood nourishes and replenishes essence. With a deficiency of Blood, the womb and the Conception and Penetrating Vessels will lack the necessary nourishment needed to nurture a fertilized egg. Women are very prone to Blood deficiency, partly due to the monthly loss of blood occurring with menstruation and partly from diet, overwork and emotional stress.

Symptoms: Blood deficiency is commonly seen in patients with amenorrhoea (a lack of periods), polycystic ovaries and Polycystic Ovary Syndrome (PCOS). Patients often have insomnia, light periods, dizziness, palpitations, a lustreless complexion, dry skin, pale lips and tongue, and a thready or fine pulse.

Case study

Irena, aged 37

PROBLEM:	**irregular menstrual cycle, peri-menopause**
METHODS TRIED	**diagnostic tests only**
TCM OBJECTIVE:	**to clear abdominal obstruction and improve ovarian function**
LENGTH OF TREATMENT:	**12 months and ongoing consultations**
OUTCOME:	**natural conception; 2 children in the long term**

Irena was 37 years old when she came to see us. She had always had an irregular menstrual cycle. It was the reason she originally went on the pill. But she had been off it for four years, in which time she had not conceived.

A diagnostic laparoscopy revealed that she had stage 1 endometriosis. One of her fallopian tubes was normal, the other had hydrosalpinx (see page 82). Her menstrual cycles were between 14 and 60 days with six to seven days of premenstrual bleeding. The blood lost was dark and clotted and she sometimes suffered from period pain. Her FSH reading was between 10.9 and 19.9 IU/L. Inhibin B and Anti-Mullerian hormone were almost undetectable. She was not considered a suitable candidate for IVF via the NHS.

TCM assessment and treatment plan

Conventional diagnosis categorized Irena's symptoms as peri-menopausal. I have seen a vast number of women with a reasonably regular menstrual cycle between the ages of 35 and 45 who also have high FSH levels. Those women are still able to get pregnant during this time. However, as their fertility has reached its peak and begins to decline as age increases, the chances of getting pregnant reduce.

Irena's tongue texture was normal, with normal coating, her pulses were normal/ wiry and there was no physical abnormality. Because she had always had irregular periods it was impossible to prejudge whether TCM might help her to achieve a pregnancy. My view was that although her endometriosis was mild, it was an indication of abdominal obstruction. A TCM programme would focus initially on clearing her abdominal environment, which would encourage her reproductive organs to function better.

During her eight-month programme of TCM treatment, Irena had three regular menstrual cycles of 26 to 28 days. She then became pregnant but miscarried shortly afterwards, at five and a half weeks. Both Irena and I were encouraged by this development and we continued with TCM for a further four months. She conceived again and remained on TCM until week 13 of her pregnancy. She was then discharged until week 36. At that point we prescribed one week's worth of herbal tablets to be taken immediately after the birth, in the hope that her uterus would recover more quickly.

A year later, while Irena was still breastfeeding, she returned to see us for advice on achieving a second pregnancy. I told her to wait until she had stopped breastfeeding and her periods had returned. We could then organize an up-to-date hormone test for her. Four months passed, with no sign of a period. We were getting worried, as we knew how irregular her periods had been before. I organized an ultrasound scan for Irena before putting her on the TCM programme, just to be on the safe side. To our mutual surprise, we found she was 18 weeks pregnant!

Irena's first birth was slightly premature, so we kept her on the TCM treatment until week 38. We suspended all acupuncture and herbal medicine at this point and expected her pregnancy to go full term. Just three days after she stopped the TCM, Irena gave birth to her second child.

Infertility patterns in men

References to fertility treatments aimed at men in China date back as far as the Sui Dynasty in AD 589. This shows that responsibility was not placed exclusively with women, but was shared between husband and wife. In China, the treatment of male infertility is generally seen as easier than that of female infertility because the male reproductive system is less complicated.

EXCESS PATTERNS

As with female infertility, male infertility is categorized into excess and deficient patterns, though a patient may be suffering from a combination of the two.

Damp-Heat

Damp-Heat in the Spleen and/or Liver, aggravated by fatty foods and alcohol, leads to Dampness or Phlegm formation in the genitals. *Yin*-deficient Heat and prolonged stagnation of *qi* and Dampness due to Spleen deficiency and Liver constraint can also cause this pattern. Dampness flows down and Damp-Heat, in particular, collects in the Liver Meridian (see page 50) and as a consequence blocks the genitals as the Liver Meridian serves the genitals.

Symptoms: Blockage of ejaculatory ducts, reduced sperm count, limited motility, a high level of abnormal sperm forms or white cell count, inflammation and itchiness around the groin or infections correspond to this condition. Men typically present with symptoms of erectile dysfunction, often in combination with a feeling of heaviness, yellow discharge from the penis, thick ejaculate, a red tongue with greasy coating and a rapid and slippery pulse.

Liver *qi* stagnation and Blood stasis

In men, Liver *qi* stagnation is often connected with an insufficiency of essence, which prevents Blood and muscles being replenished. The erection may be temporarily weak or there might be periods of impotence or premature ejaculation and the structural quality of sperm may be poor. When the Liver can no longer perform its function to supply the muscles and tendons or sinews with sufficient *qi* and Blood, it will result in blockages.

Symptoms: As the penis is regarded as the 'sinew of the Liver', erectile dysfunction, varicoceles, tenderness in the groin or blockage of the ejaculatory duct are associated with this pattern.

Blood Heat

Heat dries out fluids and Blood, causing the body to lack fluids and resulting in a low sperm count, even azoospermia. See page 106 for more information.

Symptoms: Blood Heat is commonly seen in men with a severely low sperm count or a low volume of seminal fluid. Men with Blood Heat find it difficult to get off to sleep and dream a lot. They may display red lips and a red tongue with no coating.

DEFICIENT PATTERNS

As we have seen, the basic requirements for achieving full reproductive potential in TCM is strong Kidney *jing* and a balance between Kidney *yin* and Kidney *yang*, *qi* and Blood. The causes for depletion in men are no different from depletion in women, as described above (see page 107–109).

Yin and Blood

Kidney *yin* represents the substance and storehouse of prenatal essence and energy reserve. If these reserves are exhausted without being restored, infertility will result. Blood, an aspect of *yin*, is produced by the Spleen from the food we eat, and in men is transformed into sperm.

Symptoms: A deficiency of *yin* and Blood is related to problems with sperm count and semen volume. Patients with this type usually have a high number of abnormal sperm and long-term infertility.

Yang and *qi*

Kidney *qi* is the mobilizing force that distributes *yin* and *yang* and is closely related to Kidney *yang*. *Yang* and *qi* are the motivating force behind the sperm when they break through an egg's coating and a deficiency of these affects sperm motility and ejaculation.

Symptoms: The uplifting and containing function of Kidney *qi* affects body fluids, including sperm and urine. Frequent urination is a typical symptom of Kidney *qi* deficiency, while feeling cold is the primary symptom of *yang* deficiency as *yang* warms the body. A deficiency of *qi* leads to weakness in the uplifting strength, which results in shortened erection or impotence, nightly release of semen, a low sperm count and low motility. In conjunction there is often pain in the lumbar region and knees.

PART 3

TRADITIONAL CHINESE MEDICINE AND TREATMENTS

Chapter 7

CONDITIONS AND TREATMENTS

Plants are very powerful natural medicines and have been used to heal for millennia. Every child knows that if you are stung by a stinging nettle you rub a dock leaf over the rash to soothe it – and that they are always to be found growing conveniently close to the nettles! If you have a headache, the chances are you reduce the pain by washing down some willow bark with a glass of water – although you will know it as aspirin made from salicylic acid derived from willow bark.

Every culture has distilled its own medicinal tradition from the plants that grow in the local environment. Today, the Amazonian rainforest remains probably the biggest natural pharmacy in the world.

Traditional Chinese Medicine is regarded as a complementary or alternative medicine in Western countries, yet it is one of the oldest and best-documented catalogues of remedies in the world. It is based on a sophisticated medical philosophy that uses almost 3,000 different ingredients. It is a tradition that has been developed and used over centuries and practised in China for more than 5,000 years. TCM is still the primary care choice in China and other Asian countries, although Western medicine is usually practised in parallel.

Modern Western medicine is a relatively young discipline. Its roots lie in the work of ancient physicians, such as Hippocrates (known as the father of modern medicine), and herbalists and apothecaries, such as Nicolas Culpeper, whose *Herbal* was published in 1653. These days, synthetic versions of the plants are used, made from identical chemical compounds, but in reality we are all still using plants to heal ourselves so there's nothing unorthodox about using herbal medicine.

However, TCM is a highly specialized discipline and is used in a way that is different from Western medicine. At its most basic level, Western medicine usually uses a single drug to treat a symptom; for example, an eczema cream may relieve the symptoms of eczema. However, this doesn't address the root cause of why the body is creating this skin condition. Chinese herbs are used to treat the symptoms as well as trying to rectify the underlying problem, caused either by an excess or a deficiency. If you have an excess of Heat you will be treated by cooling herbs, if you have Damp you will be given herbs to disperse it, if you have Blood stasis the herbs prescribed will clear and move the Blood, and so on.

Clinical research has discovered that certain Chinese herbs have strong anti-oestrogenic and anti-androgen properties so are invaluable in the treatment of fertility.

HOW LONG DOES TCM TAKE TO WORK?

The time it takes for Chinese herbs to have a healing effect on the body will differ from person to person, depending on the constitution of the individual, the problem they have and the way they respond to the treatment. That is why, at my clinic, we always recommend that those who would like to benefit from TCM should try the treatment several months *before* starting any assisted fertility treatment such as IUI, IVF or ICSI.

TCM treatments

An individual's TCM treatment plan can normally be decided during the course of a diagnosis consultation. The patient's symptoms and signs are analysed and summarized, together with their constitution, pulse, tongue, lifestyle, diet and environment. (For more about this, see pages 31–33.)

TCM regards the human body as an integral whole, with special emphasis on achieving internal harmony and balance in the body. But the external environment of the body is also important, so climatic, geographic, social and other environmental factors that have an impact on physical and mental wellbeing are taken into consideration as well.

Sometimes the same treatment programme is used for different types of problems in the same patient or, alternatively, different treatment programmes may be used, depending on the person's TCM 'type' (see pages 117–135). It is common for a person to be prescribed several different remedies during the course of treatment as the organs change and respond to the support being given.

There are always two major aspects to an individual treatment plan. The practitioner needs to consider which symptoms imply *excess* and which show *deficiency* (see pages 104–112) in the organs of the body.

Excesses show in the form of:

- Blood stasis (see pages 118–120)
- Excessive Liver *qi* stagnation (see pages 120–122)
- Excessive Phlegm-Damp (see pages 125–126)
- Excessive Damp-Heat (see pages 126–128)
- Excessive Blood Heat (see pages 128–132)

Deficiencies show in the form of:

- Blood (and *qi*) deficiency (see pages 132–133)
- Kidney *yin* deficiency (see pages 133–135)
- Kidney *yang* deficiency (see pages 135–136)

Where there is an excess, the treatment needs to clear, clean, move away or expel the cause and the symptoms. It is like renovating a house: one room may need just a new coat of paint and a new set of curtains, whereas other rooms need to be completely stripped down and renovated before redecoration can take place. It all depends on the individual case.

The majority of patients who undergo IVF treatment need several months of TCM to get the body ready or in better condition. In our clinic, of the patients who follow our recommended treatment programme and become pregnant, 39 per cent achieve pregnancy within six months, a further 46 per cent within one year and 15 per cent conceive after one to two years. Of course, treatment takes longer for some than for others, it all depends on the patient, the nature of her body and the way she responds. Treatment is much quicker for patients who only need the clearing of an excessive unhealthy type, than for those who need clearing, then tonifying.

On average, it takes between nine months and one year for our patients to become pregnant, and an average of three courses of treatment. Of course, for those who do not have fertility problems, the result may be quicker. It is important to have realistic expectations of how long the process may take, otherwise you will put yourself under undue pressure, which will not help the process.

TONIFYING

'Tonifying' has a very precise meaning in TCM: it is the process of replenishing *qi*, Blood, *yin* and *yang* in the body.

What TCM type are you?

One of the ways in which TCM differs so much from Western medicine is that TCM treats the person as a whole, including both the physical and emotional aspects of the body. The person is treated as an individual, rather than the sum of their physical symptoms. We do not concentrate solely on the physical indicators to diagnose the problem. What matters is your own unique composition, so that any treatment can be tailor-made to suit you.

That means, if your sister, brother or friend is also undergoing treatment, don't expect yours to be the same as theirs. It is not a case of 'one size fits all'. You may be related by genetics or blood, you may have a similar underlying condition, but if you have a totally different pattern or type, your treatment will be different.

In TCM we determine your type by analysing the signals your body displays. The clues build a picture of what imbalances are causing your system to malfunction. Like fine-tuning a piano, it takes sensitivity and patience to listen to and identify the cause of the problem but the end result is harmonious.

The philosophy behind TCM suggests that you are born with a certain constitution, which predisposes you to be a certain TCM type. However, your lifestyle and emotions can affect your type. For example, living life too hard or carrying a lot of internalized rage can lead to the body being out of balance.

We can identify their main type by asking patients a few simple questions, and by observing their tongue, pulse and general constitution. If you answer the questions below you should be able to identify your own type, which will help you to understand my guidelines for diet, herbs and acupuncture treatment in the sections that follow. It will also prepare you well if you decide to have professional TCM treatment.

Don't be confused if you seem to fall into more than one type – it's perfectly possible to suffer from both Damp-Heat and Liver *qi* stagnation, it just takes a little more effort to 'fine tune' your diagnosis. If you find you have answered 'yes' to more questions in one of the categories than in the others – then this is likely to be your dominant type.

SELF-PRESCRIPTION OF HERBS

I always stress to my patients that they should not be tempted to self-prescribe herbs or to buy over-the-counter remedies without taking professional advice. The herbs are very powerful and can cause damage if taken inappropriately – especially when trying to become pregnant.

BLOOD STASIS

Blood stasis is characterized by the stagnation of Blood circulation or the coagulation of Blood that has leaked or been forced from the vessels that should contain it. This is usually due to stagnation of vital energy, a deficiency of vital energy and Blood, Blood Heat or as a result of being unable to fully recover from a trauma such as surgery or injury.

Answer 'Yes' or 'No' to the questions below and add up your score at the end.

Women:

Do you suffer from painful periods?
Do you need painkillers before or during your period?
Is your period often late?
Do you suffer from intermittent bleeding or spotting between normal periods?
Do you experience a relief from menstrual pain after the discharge of clots?
Have you ever been diagnosed with ovarian cysts or endometriomas?
Do you have scarce and purplish, dark menstrual discharge with clots?
Do you have sharp, fixed, stabbing menstrual pain, which is worse with pressure?
Do you suffer from abdominal pain that starts after ovulation?
Does your basal temperature not drop on Day 1 of your cycle?
Have you ever been diagnosed with endometriosis?
Have you experienced an ectopic pregnancy in the past?

Men:

Do you have painful testicles?
Do you have a heavy or dragging feeling in the testicular area?
Have you been diagnosed with varicocele?
Do you feel abdominal discomfort or pain?

Both:

Do your hands and feet often feel cold?
Do you experience periodic pins and needles or numbness in the limbs?
Does your tongue look purple in colour?
Do you have a tendency to varicose veins?
Number of questions answered 'Yes':
Number of questions answered 'No':
The relevance of your score: If you answered 'Yes' to more than half the relevant questions above, then it is likely that your type is Blood stasis. Turn to page 137 for a treatment plan.

Case study

Grace, aged 37

PROBLEM:	**PCOS; trying to conceive for 5 years**
METHODS TRIED:	**2 IUI cycles, 3 IVF cycles, ICSI**
TCM OBJECTIVE:	**to improve *qi* and Blood, and to regulate the menstrual cycle**
LENGTH OF TREATMENT:	**5 months, initially**
OUTCOME:	**natural conception; 3 children in the long term**

Grace came to see us at the age of 37. She and her husband had been trying to conceive for five years without success. She had undergone a laparoscopy, ultrasound scan and hormone tests at the beginning of their fertility investigations, which confirmed she was suffering from Polycystic Ovary Syndrome (PCOS). Her menstrual cycle showed typical signs of PCOS, as it varied between 45 and 75 days. Her husband's semen analyses were all within normal range. The couple had undergone two IUI and three IVF cycles and a final ICSI cycle, but had failed to conceive.

TCM assessment and treatment plan

Grace complained of painful periods during which she would lose a lot of dark-coloured blood, with clots. She had typical symptoms of Blood stasis and her tongue was lightly pink with purplish spots, like pin points (this colouration is the result of poor Blood circulation causing a tendency to cyanosis). Her pulses were deep and fine, which indicated the Blood flow was low.

Typically for someone with PCOS, Grace would produce lots of follicles under the follicle stimulating injection, but most of them were underdeveloped and immature. This is due to reduced blood flow to the ovaries. In Grace's case, 12 to 15 eggs were collected, but fewer than half of them resulted in embryos. On her second IVF cycle, none were fertilized at all.

Her treatment programme was initially designed to improve her Blood circulation. After four weeks of herbal medication, the appearance of her tongue had changed from pale and resembling pin points to normal red with slight 'tooth marks' on both sides of the tongue. Her pulse was still deep and thin, which told me it was time to add some herbs to the formula to tonify *qi*.

By her third month of TCM treatment, Grace's cycle was at the 70-day point. I suggested that in her case it might be good idea to have a pregnancy test before continuing with further TCM, as the treatment strategy would be different if she had become pregnant. She took the test, which confirmed that she *was* pregnant. We continued TCM treatment until the third month of her pregnancy.

After giving birth to her son naturally, she returned to see us again. The couple now have three children, all conceived naturally.

LIVER *QI* STAGNATION

Liver *qi* stagnation is when *qi* is unable to flow freely through the body and the flow of vital energy is disrupted. Stagnation in certain areas can lead to local tissue and organ dysfunction. It is often caused by emotional trauma and the main symptoms are usually associated with the menstrual cycle, local swelling or pain and a lack of coordination between vital energy and Blood, which leads to the dysfunction of the body.

Answer 'Yes' or 'No' to the questions below and add up your score at the end.

Women:

Do you suffer from premenstrual tension?
Are your periods a few days early or few days late (slightly irregular)?
Do you suffer from premenstrual breast distension or sore breasts?
Do you feel emotional before your periods?
Does your follicular phase (see pages 65–66) last longer than 14 days?
Does your temperature oscillate widely in the luteal phase (see page 66)?
Do you have nipple discharge?
Do you feel abdominal discomfort or pain during ovulation?
Do you have sore or lumpy breasts?
Do you notice your stools are much looser during your periods?
Do you find it difficult to cope with your swollen breasts before your period?

Men:

Do you suffer from short-temperedness or impatience?
Do you feel abdominal discomfort or pain?
Do you have loose stools?
Do you have weak erections or a partial inability to ejaculate?

Both:

Are you prone to feel irritable, depressed or moody?
Do you sigh frequently?
Do you have a bloated stomach?
Do you feel a sensation of obstruction in the throat?
Do you suffer from irritable bowel syndrome?
Do you suffer from low libido?
Have you been diagnosed with unexplained infertility?
Number of questions answered 'Yes':

Number of questions answered 'No':

The relevance of your score: If you answered 'Yes' to more than half the relevant questions above, then it is likely that your type is Liver *qi* stagnation. Turn to page 140 for a treatment plan.

Case study

Karla, aged 44

PROBLEM:	**trying to conceive for 4 years**
METHODS TRIED:	**natural conception**
TCM OBJECTIVE:	**to eliminate Liver *qi* stagnation**
LENGTH OF TREATMENT:	**6 months**
OUTCOME:	**improved ovarian function; a son**

Karla was 40 when she became pregnant with her daughter. Two years later she conceived again, but miscarried at 11 weeks. She turned to TCM at the age of 44 years, 6 months.

Karla had undergone two laparoscopies to remove ovarian cysts before conceiving her first child, and had laser treatment for endometriosis. All her ovarian reserve tests such as FSH, LH, oestradiol, prolactin and tests for ovarian fertility potential, such as Anti-Mullerian hormone and inhibin B, were all within reasonably normal range despite her age. An ultrasound scan and hysteroscopy were also normal and her husband's semen analysis did not show any abnormality.

TCM assessment and treatment plan

Karla had an excellent ovarian reserve, which indicated that she still had a good fertility potential. Her menstrual cycle had been regular at 28 days in the past, but had become slightly erratic in recent years – between 25 and 30 days – and bleeding varied between light or heavy. She also experienced headaches before her periods. Other symptoms included two to three days of postmenstrual or premenstrual bleeding and some lower backache and lower abdominal pain. She had a normal-looking tongue and her pulses were wiry and fine.

There appeared to be typical symptoms of *qi* stagnation. The physical and psychological symptoms appear and disappear according to the fluctuation of *qi* flow. Stagnant Liver *qi* disrupts all organs along the Liver Meridian pathway, hence she suffered from headaches and also complained of occasional painful periods. In peri-menopausal women, decreased oestrogen production may cause Kidney *yin* to become deficient and less able to harmonize the function of the other organs. This is why she had lower backache.

The treatment principle for Karla was to eliminate the Liver *qi* stagnation and harmonize the Liver and Kidney function so that Karla's normal ovarian function could be improved. This would help her to achieve a pregnancy. Karla had been on TCM treatment for three months, during which she reported that she no longer suffered from headaches, and discovered that she was pregnant.

Karla continued with TCM treatment until she was 13 weeks pregnant and then she was discharged. She gave birth to a healthy little boy.

LIVER *QI* STAGNATION AND EXCESSIVE HEAT

A diagnosis of Liver *qi* stagnation and Heat is often linked to emotional anger. However, as you near the peri-menopause the body naturally tends more towards Heat due to the reduced production of oestrogen; your hair, skin and eyes feel drier and you may suffer vaginal dryness. TCM seeks to restore coolness and fluidity to Heat sufferers by increasing *yin* (cooling, nourishing and moistening) functions.

People who work too hard, are constantly under stress and eat on the go often display signs of Liver *qi* stagnation and Heat, so lifestyle changes are important to restore soothing calm.

Answer 'Yes' or 'No' to the questions below and add up your score at the end.

Women:

Is your basal temperature above 36.6°C in the follicular phase (see pages 65–66)?
Do you have an unstable follicular phase with temperature variations of more than 0.2–0.3°C?
Do you often feel hot and sweaty before periods?
Is your menstrual cycle prone to be shorter than normal?
Do you notice incessant dripping of blood after periods?
Do you have fluctuating FSH levels?
Do you often suffer from headaches before your period starts?
Have you experienced ovulation before egg collection takes place during IVF?
Do you suffer from unexplained high prolactin levels?

Men:

Do you often feel hot and sweaty?
Do you often experience premature ejaculation?

Both:

Do you find it difficult to get to sleep?
Do you feel angry easily and with little provocation?

Do you suffer from an overactive thyroid gland?

Do you suffer from constipation?

Do you feel thirsty often and drink a lot?

Do you suffer from headaches and dislike the sunlight?

Number of questions answered 'Yes':

Number of questions answered 'No':

The relevance of your score: If you answered 'Yes' to more than half the relevant questions above, then it is likely that your type is Liver *qi* stagnation and excessive Heat. Turn to page 143 for a treatment plan.

Case study

Carole, aged 38

PROBLEM:	**unexplained infertility**
METHODS TRIED:	**3 ICSI cycles, HUMIRA injection to decrease NK cells**
TCM OBJECTIVE:	**to clear Liver *qi* stagnation and reduce excessive heat**
LENGTH OF TREATMENT:	**6 months**
OUTCOME:	**natural conception; a son**

Carole was 38 and her husband was 37 years old. They had been diagnosed with unexplained infertility and chose to seek help through TCM after they had failed their third ICSI cycle with HUMIRA injections (see box, below).

Carole underwent some investigative tests, including laparoscopy and a dye test, hysteroscopy and ovarian reserve test, all of which showed no signs of abnormality apart from raised FSH levels – which reached 16.9 at some points. She also had raised levels of NK cells. Her husband had four semen analyses, all of which were within normal range.

HUMIRA

HUMIRA (Human Monoclonal Antibody in Rheumatoid Arthritis) is a chemical blocking agent, used to block the effect of TNF (tumour necrosis factor) – which sounds rather alarming, but in effect it reduces the level of inflammation in autoimmune cells when the body is under threat. It is most often used to treat forms of arthritis, Crohn's disease and asthma. It is also used by some fertility clinics to reduce the level and impact of natural killer (NK) cells, which some believe will 'attack' the unborn foetus (see page 96 for more about NK cells). HUMIRA is not licensed for use in reproductive medicine because not enough is known about its effects on the foetus and the unborn child. Nevertheless, some women will opt for the treatment if their fertility clinic supports its use.

TCM assessment and treatment plan

Carole's raised FSH indicated that she did have an ovarian reserve. She had undergone three ICSI cycles. The first seemed to respond well: nine eggs were collected and seven became embryos. However, most of the eggs were of poor quality. During the following two ICSI cycles it became clear that her ovary function was worsening and she couldn't produce an egg that was healthy enough to achieve fertilization. No matter how much work you put in to assisting implantation (such as using HUMIRA injections), the quality of the embryo remains the primary key to success.

TCM diagnosis showed that Carol's Liver *qi* had transformed and showed symptoms of Heat. Her menstrual cycle was slightly short: between 23 and 25 days, with three or four days of bleeding. She complained of PMS and frequent migraines, and suffered from lots of headaches. She felt thirsty all the time and her tongue was red with a thin coating. Her pulses were wiry and aggressive. All the above symptoms are typical of Liver *qi* stagnation transformed into Heat, which had affected her immunological system (and may be associated with raised NK cell levels).

After taking TCM herbs for six weeks, Carole discovered she was pregnant, but miscarried at six weeks. Carole was not overwhelmingly upset by the outcome as finally there was something to show for her three years of ICSI cycles. I advised Carole to use contraception for at least three months, to allow more time to help her to improve her ovary function, which would result in better egg quality. She remained on TCM for a further six months. She had no more headaches, her thirst reduced and she had fewer symptoms of PMS. We agreed she should come off the Pill, and she became pregnant again.

Carole was concerned that the previous pregnancy might have been lost because of her history of raised NK cell levels. She returned to her fertility clinic for tests during her second pregnancy. However, the blood test reported that her NK cell level was now almost undetectable. The pregnancy went very well after we discharged her from our clinic at 13 weeks. She went on to give birth to a healthy little boy.

I would not dream of taking all the credit for helping Carole to achieve her pregnancy and live birth as there is insufficient clinical evidence to prove that the TCM had lowered her NK cell level. Also, she was having HUMIRA injections during the last two ICSI cycles, which may have also had an impact. However, I am certain that the work we did to clear her internal toxicity, balance her internal organs and support the internal system to enable it to work harmoniously will have definitely helped Carole to improve her ovarian function and benefited the quality of her eggs. Whether the symptoms of Liver *qi* stagnation transferring into Heat are connected in some way with the incidence of raised NK cells is something I wish to investigate in more depth.

PHLEGM-DAMP

Phlegm-Damp people have systems that are, literally, clogged with Damp-producing substances and may notice fluid retention and swelling. They are prone to allergies and eczema and if this is your type, you may suffer from catarrh and excess mucus. You may also crave sweet, fatty foods. Damp type is stubborn. It can take a little longer to clear from the system and a sustained change in diet is often required.

Answer 'Yes' or 'No' to the questions below and add up your score at the end.

Women:
Do you notice your menstrual cycles are longer than 30 days?
Have you been diagnosed with polycystic ovaries or PCOS?
Do you often have vaginal discharges?
Is your menstrual blood brown in colour?
Do you have heavy or sticky discharge?

Men:
Do you suffer from low sperm motility?
Do you have a high number of abnormal forms in your semen samples?

Both:
Do you feel you need more than eight hours sleep at night?
Do you feel sleepy or sleep deeply?
Do feel heavy or fuzzy headed?
Do you still feel tired in the morning even after a good night's sleep?
Do you have a thick coating on your tongue?
Do you have soft stools or easily get diarrhoea?
Are you slightly overweight or obese?
Do your limbs feel heavy?
Do you suffer from nausea?
Have you been diagnosed with insulin resistance?
Have you been diagnosed with a rising insulin level?
Number of questions answered 'Yes':
Number of questions answered 'No':

The relevance of your score: If you answered 'Yes' to more than half the relevant questions above, then it is likely that your type is Phlegm-Damp. Turn to page 144 for a treatment plan.

Case study

Christophe, aged 32

PROBLEM:	**low sperm count, low motility**
TCM OBJECTIVE:	**to clear Phlegm-Damp**
LENGTH OF TREATMENT:	**3 months**
OUTCOME:	**natural conception; a daughter**

Christophe was just 32 when he came to see me, and as soon as he walked into my room I could see that he was suffering. He was slightly overweight, tired, hot and sweaty. During the consultation he said he slept a lot but remained very tired, and had loose bowel movements three to four times a day. He also had a thick coating on his tongue.

Christophe had a low sperm count (less than 1 million per ml), a low motility level of less than 10 per cent and 99 per cent of his sperm were of abnormal form.

TCM assessment and treatment plan
My main focus was to clear the Phlegm-Damp from his system so that the normal flow of *qi* and Blood could resume healthily.

Christophe was on herbal treatments for 12 weeks. And as well as treating him with acupuncture, we used moxibustion heat treatments (see pages 233–234) once the Phlegm-Damp had reduced, at a later stage. His tiredness reduced and, significantly, his bowel movements became normal – reducing to just once a day. His semen sample improved too. Soon afterwards his wife became pregnant naturally and they had a healthy girl.

DAMP-HEAT

When Damp stays in the body for a long period of time without being successfully treated it can easily develop into Damp-Heat. Eventually the Damp and Heat builds up in the lower part of the body, resulting in an abdominal inflammation and disturbing the lower part of the body's normal function. Often we need to clear the Damp and Heat obstruction so we can allow a healthy Blood supply to circulate properly in the abdomen, where it can deliver to the uterus and ovaries.

Answer 'Yes' or 'No' to the questions below and add up your score at the end.

Women:

Do you easily get urine infections or cystitis symptoms?

Have you had Pelvic Inflammatory Disease (PID) in the past?

Have you been diagnosed as having damaged fallopian tubes?

Have you experienced a miscarriage due to chromosome abnormality?

Have you been diagnosed as having endometriosis?

Have you experienced an ectopic pregnancy?

Do you have yellow or sticky discharge?

Men:

Have you ever experienced a rise in white blood cells in your semen sample?

Have you had swollen testicles in the past?

Do you suffer from itching or a rash in the groin area?

Both:

Do you need to get up at night to pass urine?

Do you have oily skin?

Have you ever experienced eczema?

Do you often experience puffy hands and feet, particularly in summer?

Do you have a thick and yellow coating on your tongue?

Do you suffer from yeast infections?

Number of questions answered 'Yes':

Number of questions answered 'No':

The relevance of your score: If you answered 'Yes' to more than half the relevant questions above, then it is likely that your type is Damp-Heat. Turn to page 147 for a treatment plan.

Case study

Julia, aged 35

PROBLEM:	**trying to conceive for 4½ years**
METHODS TRIED:	**IUI, 3 IVF cycles, FET**
TCM OBJECTIVE:	**to clear the abdomen of Damp and Heat**
LENGTH OF TREATMENT:	**6 months**
OUTCOME:	**natural conception; 4 children in the long term**

Julia first came to see me at the age of 35. She had been trying to conceive for four and a half years. She had previously been for a hysterosalpingogram (HSG) test, but was shown to have no significant problem. However, an investigative laparoscopy showed a twisted and narrowed fallopian tube, which was thought to be contributing to her fertility issues.

Since then she had tried IUI, known as 'artificial insemination', but there had been no pregnancy. She then underwent three cycles of IVF treatment – also without success. Interestingly, seven eggs were collected during each cycle, and as many as six fertilized every time. She also went through a frozen embryo transfer (FET). All had failed to achieve a pregnancy, but no one had been able to tell her why. Her menstrual cycle, at 26 to 27 days long, was reasonably normal – so what was the problem?

TCM assessment and treatment plan

During the initial TCM consultation, Julia complained that her bowel movements were very loose (two to three times a day) and mentioned that she suffered from chronic cystitis and thrush. These symptoms suggest a person's abdominal environment is not very healthy and told me that there was too much Damp and Heat in her body. So initially that is what we focused on – just using the herbs to clear the Damp and Heat. The result was amazing, really. She became pregnant just two months after starting treatment.

Clearly, in Julia's case, her problems conceiving had nothing at all to do with the narrow tube, or egg quality, or a stressful lifestyle. She had been through all those IVFs, and every time, the eggs matured and fertilized into embryos. However, the implantation in her uterus never took place. By clearing her abdominal environment of all the Damp and Heat, her blood was able to flow more healthily and circulate to her reproductive system so it began to function normally, allowing the implantation to take place.

I prepared some herbal medicine for Julia to take after her baby was born that would make it easier for her to conceive the next time. When her baby was six months old she came back to the clinic as she wanted to have another baby. Within two months she conceived again. She went on to have four children.

THRUSH

Thrush is thought to have a possible link with a history of Pelvic Inflammatory Disease (PID). In TCM we see it as Damp and Heat irritating the abdominal and pelvic environment. Changing your diet to reduce your intake of yeast products, dairy products and sugar will help to reduce the recurrence of thrush to a certain extent, but is unlikely to clear it out of the body. The beauty of the herbs is that they will go deep down to clear the environment systemically.

BLOOD HEAT

Most people whose type is Blood Heat are associated with a certain gene or constitution, but a diet that is hot and spicy can often increase the symptoms. If the person only needs treatment for cooling of the Blood, recovery can be quick and easy. However, when there is a need to restore fluids in the body too, this can sometimes take longer to achieve. It is rather like the difference between filling a bath with the taps on full and with partially blocked taps. It will take much longer to fill up the bath if the tap cannot be fully opened and the water is coming through at a trickle. A sensible lifestyle, combined with carefully selected therapeutic treatment and nourishment can often correct and improve this condition.

Answer 'Yes' or 'No' to the questions below and add up your score at the end.

Women:

Do you have a very short menstrual cycle?
Do you notice your menstrual discharge is purplish-red and thin?
Do you notice your periods are heavy?
Do you respond too fast to the follicle stimulating drugs during IVF?
Have you experienced ovulation before the egg collection in IVF?
Have you experienced poor response to the drugs during an IVF cycle despite your hormone tests being reasonably normal?
Have you experienced heavy bleeding from an early miscarriage?

Men:

Have you been diagnosed with azoospermia or a severely low sperm count although your male hormone test is normal?

Both:

Do you sometimes have haemorrhoids (piles)?
Do you ever feel your heartbeat rising or palpitations?
Do you notice your lips are red and dry?
Do you have disturbed sleep and dream often?
Do you notice your dreams are often violent?
Is your tongue red, slim and without a coating?
Do you have red cheeks, particularly in the afternoon?
Do you tend to be slightly underweight even though you eat a lot?
Do you feel hot most of the time?
Do you have dizzy spells sometimes?
Do you easily get nosebleeds?
Number of questions answered 'Yes':
Number of questions answered 'No':

Case study

Judy, aged 35/Adam, aged 36

PROBLEMS:	**trying to conceive for 3 years/severely low sperm count**
METHODS TRIED:	**4 ICSI cycles, one of which used donor sperm**
TCM OBJECTIVE:	**to clear Blood Heat and improve Blood flow**
LENGTH OF TREATMENT:	**2 years**
OUTCOME:	**natural conception; 2 children in the long term**

Judy and her husband, Adam, had been trying to conceive for three years. Her husband had a very low sperm count of only 1–2 million per ml, and less than 10 per cent motility. ICSI treatment is always the first option in the case of male infertility problems, because the sperm can be selected and then injected into the egg, external to the body. They had been through four ICSI cycles before coming to see me, and in the most recent ICSI cycle, donor sperm was used. This told me that their consultant believed male infertility to be the root cause of their problem.

TCM assessment

Judy had responded well to IVF stimulation drugs and had produced an excellent number of follicles, with as many as 15 to 17 eggs being collected at a time, about ten of which were suitable to use for ICSI. However, only two or three were fertilized each time, which was a very low result. Interestingly, when the couple used donor sperm, the results were even worse. Of ten eggs collected, only one was fertilized. The donor sperm had made no difference. This told me clearly that ICSI was not overcoming the main problem – so the problem was *not* only male infertility.

None of Judy's investigative tests had revealed any problems. Her tubal patency test result was fine and she had no hormonal problems. She was only 35 – which was quite young in terms of reproductive age. Her cycle was very regular: every 30 days.

I started looking into Judy's overall reproductive system. The woman's ovaries need to be in good shape to respond effectively to fertility drugs. Not only does the egg quality need to be good, but also the abdominal environment needs to be right for fertilization and for carrying the pregnancy. In Judy's case there were signs that there was room for improvement.

Judy told me that she suffered from very painful periods and needed painkillers. I began to pay attention to the possibility of Blood stasis. Her tongue was incredibly red – purple-red, with no coating. That means the person has Heat in the Blood and also indicates some level of Blood stasis. Her pulse was very weak, 'choppy' and hesitant. That was further evidence of Blood stasis and told me that her Blood supply was not flowing properly. Although a weak Blood supply may sometimes indicate deficiency problems too, as she was very young I felt this was unlikely.

TCM treatment plan

My first priority was to clear the Heat and to get the Blood flowing more healthily. Judy smoked. I asked her to stop. She did. She drank 14 units a week – I asked her to cut down to no more than two units – and to stop all together if she could. Within two weeks she told me that her skin had improved and that her abdomen did not feel so windy. Over the next 11 months she visited me every fortnight. I altered the herbs according to her symptoms. Gradually her condition improved, her tongue was less red, her pulse was stronger and we were able to get her cycle down to 27 to 29 days rather than 30.

Once Judy's ovulation cycle and overall condition were stable, I asked to treat Adam. He had similar symptoms to Judy: a dark red tongue (which may have related to their similar diet) and a very choppy pulse – as if the Blood was not flowing smoothly. Adam drank 12 to 14 units of alcohol (lager and red wine) a week. He was also slightly overweight – so I told him to stop drinking completely. They were a very nice and determined couple who did everything I asked.

My intention was to improve Adam's sperm quality in preparation for IVF. Very quickly, his semen analysis showed an increased sperm count of 10 million per ml and 35 to 46 per cent motility. Within two months, to everyone's surprise, they conceived by themselves, naturally.

I never saw them again, but 18 months later I received a Christmas card to say they had conceived another baby – *without me*! She said, *'I think you probably fixed me for good'*!

This is something that I see quite a lot. Once the woman has had one baby, the couple is able to conceive more easily the second time around. They had no need of IVF at all. It was an amazing outcome for them, and very satisfying for me, too.

When both the man and woman have potential problems I always concentrate on the woman first, because the woman's reproductive system is the more complicated and takes longer to be corrected. I will treat the man once the woman's health is rebalanced and a regular cycle is established. That way the TCM process is more efficient overall.

The truth is that so long as men can produce sperm, no matter what other problems are present, it is not too difficult to deal with. A woman's reproductive system is more complex to treat, compounded by the fact that inevitably, over time, there will be a dramatic decline in her ability to conceive.

The interesting lesson to learn from this case is, don't assume that your partner's low sperm count is the sole reason why you cannot conceive. Even if a woman's medical test results suggest that everything is in working order, there may well be aspects of her diet and lifestyle that are contributing to the problem; or there may be an underlying constitutional issue.

BLOOD AND *QI* DEFICIENCY

This is a condition of general debility caused by profuse bleeding and lack of vitality in the internal organs, especially those of the abdomen. This leads to interference in the production of Blood and essence. Deficient people tend to be pale, especially under their nails, inside the eyelids and on their lips. Their menstrual blood may also be pale, rather than bright red.

Answer 'Yes' or 'No' to the questions below and add up your score at the end.

Women:
Do you get dizzy or suffer from light headaches during periods?
Are your periods often late?
Are your periods prone to be light or scanty?
Do you have pain after your period?
Have tests shown you have a low level of the hormone oestradiol during Days 2 to 4 of your menstrual cycle?

Both:
Are you prone to waking up early in the morning?
Do you suffer from disturbed sleep?
Do you suffer from dryness, such as dry skin and hair?
Are your nails dry and brittle?
Do you suffer from anxiety?
Are you prone to hysteria or extreme neurosis?
Do you sometimes feel palpitations?
Do you notice you have a pale complexion?
Do you suffer from fatigue or tiredness?
Number of questions answered 'Yes':
Number of questions answered 'No':
The relevance of your score: If you answered 'Yes' to more than half the relevant questions above, then it is likely that your type is Blood and *qi* deficiency. Turn to page 155 for a treatment plan.

Case study

Ron, aged 30

PROBLEM:	**anti-sperm antibodies**
METHODS TRIED:	**IVF, ICSI**
TCM OBJECTIVE:	**to improve Spleen *qi***
LENGTH OF TREATMENT:	**5 months**
OUTCOME:	**ICSI assisted conception; a son**

Ron came to see me because results of a Mixed Antiglobulin Reaction (MAR) test suggested that he had developed anti-sperm antibodies, measured at 80 per cent. Apart from this, his sperm count, motility, progression and abnormal forms were all within the normal range. He and his wife, Sara, had had one attempt at IVF and one of ICSI, with one egg being fertilized each time, but no pregnancies had resulted.

TCM assessment and treatment plan

Ron had had a hernia repair operation five years earlier and it's possible that this operation may have disrupted the healthy functioning of his testes.

He felt tired, had a fine, slippery pulse and a normal tongue with a slightly white and greasy coating – classic signs of insufficient Spleen *qi*. We needed to restore the blood flow to the testes, dispel the Damp that had accumulated and energize the vital *qi* and Blood.

After five months of taking TCM herbal teas, another MAR test showed that Ron's sperm binding percentage had reduced to below 25 per cent. This was very good news. I advised them to try another ICSI cycle and five out of six eggs were fertilized. The couple went on to have a son. Ron's overall health is now much improved and his sleeplessness is down to his baby, not his lack of Spleen *qi*.

KIDNEY *YIN* DEFICIENCY

A deficiency of Kidney *yin* may occur in those who are born with a weak constitution or may also develop in those who have been 'overdoing things', therefore depleting their Kidneys. This usually leads to abnormal hyper-function of the Kidney.

Answer 'Yes' or 'No' to the questions below and add up your score at the end.

Women:

Do you have little or no clear, stretchy cervical mucus secretion during the follicular phase (see pages 65–66)?
Do you have delayed periods with scanty bleeding and light-coloured blood?

Men:

Do you have a low sperm count?

Do you have scanty thick seminal fluid?

Both:

Do you have a flushed complexion or feel hot in the afternoon?

Do you suffer from night sweats?

Do you suffer from constipation?

Do you have a dry mouth or throat?

Do you feel slightly thirsty in the evening?

Do you feel thirsty, but prefer hot or warm drinks?

Do you have a feverish sensation in your chest, palms and soles?

Do you tend to be slightly underweight even though you eat a lot?

Do you have no tongue coating?

Number of questions answered 'Yes':

Number of questions answered 'No':

The relevance of your score: If you answered 'Yes' to more than half the relevant questions above, then it is likely that your type is Kidney *yin* deficiency. Turn to page 158 for a treatment plan.

Case study

Peter, aged 30

PROBLEM:	**severely low sperm motility**
METHODS TRIED:	**IVF**
TCM OBJECTIVE:	**to boost Kidney *yin***
LENGTH OF TREATMENT:	**6 months**
OUTCOME:	**natural conception; a son**

Peter had low sperm motility problems. His sperm count was normal but only 1 per cent were actively moving forwards. Despite this his wife had become pregnant naturally but had then miscarried. They decided to try IVF. She then suffered an ectopic pregnancy following an IVF cycle. Two and a half years later they came to me to try TCM.

TCM assessment and treatment plan

Peter's blood pressure was high, he had poor sleep patterns, his complexion was flushed and purplish-red and he had a fine pulse. This indicated a Kidney *yin* deficiency, which was unable to harmonize the raised Heat, so my first job was to boost his Kidney *yin*.

Nourishing the kidney took several months of herbal treatment but after six months his sperm motility had improved from 1 per cent to 46 per cent and the couple became pregnant naturally. They are now parents to a healthy son.

KIDNEY *YANG* DEFICIENCY

In TCM Kidneys have a warming and flowing function. Deficiency of Kidney *yang* means that there is a deficiency in the flow of Blood and *qi* to the body's organs, and that they are underperforming.

These symptoms may also appear in women who suffer from Cold in the uterus (see pages 153–154), which may occur following birth or miscarriage.

Answer 'Yes' or 'No' to the questions below and add up your score at the end.

Women:
Is your Basal Body Temperature lower than 36.0°C on Day 1 of your cycle?
Does your Basal Body Temperature rise too slowly after ovulation? (See pages 67–71.)
Does your temperature in the luteal phase (see page 66) rise less than 0.2°C, or can the rise not be sustained for at least 12 days?
Do you have delayed periods and scanty menstruation with light-coloured blood?

Men:
Do you have watery seminal fluid?
Do you often experience premature ejaculation?
Do you suffer from impotence?

Both:
Do you dislike cold or suffer from cold limbs?
Do you have loose or pale stools?
Do you have frequent clear urination?
Do you suffer from an underactive thyroid?
Do you have a wet tongue coating?
Do you get tired quickly?
Do you suffer from lower backache?
Number of questions answered 'Yes':
Number of questions answered 'No':
The relevance of your score: If you answered 'Yes' to more than half the relevant questions above, then it is likely that your type is Kidney *yang* deficiency. Turn to page 164 for a treatment plan.

Case study

Karen, aged 42/Tony, aged 42

PROBLEM: **unexplained secondary infertility/severely low sperm count with decreased motility**

METHODS TRIED: **natural conception**

TCM OBJECTIVE: **to increase Blood flow to the uterus**

LENGTH OF TREATMENT: **9 months**

OUTCOME: **natural conception; a son**

Karen's first son was conceived and born naturally when she was aged 40, after trying for a year. One year later, she and her husband, Tony, began trying for a second baby, but after 15 months of trying unsuccessfully, they had begun to feel time was running out. Karen's age was a factor working against them so they went straight to a fertility clinic, where the consultant ran ultrasound scans, monitored Karen's menstrual cycle and checked her blood pressure level, but no obvious problems were found. Tony's sperm count was found to be very low, with decreased motility. The fertility specialist advised them to consider ICSI and IVF but they couldn't cope with the personal pressure of facing this at the time.

TCM assessment and treatment plan

When Karen and Tony came to my clinic I felt confident I could treat Tony. His sperm count, quality and motility returned to normal after just two months of treatment – he was amazed.

I knew that it might take longer to discover what wasn't working well for Karen. Her fertility specialist had been very negative about her age and suggested that she had left it too late to conceive again.

I prescribed Karen with herbs that were intended to increase Kidney *yang*, which helps to move the Blood flow to the uterus and improve egg quality. This is vital at the age of 42, when the quality of viable eggs is diminishing. Karen persevered with treatment for nine months, coming to see me every month for acupuncture and assessment of her progress. I was very impressed with how calm she remained. She was a therapist, so understood that a relaxed mind can help the body to function well.

To everyone's surprise, Karen then discovered she was pregnant. She had conceived naturally. She was nine weeks into the pregnancy before she realized, having had a small bleed the previous month, which she assumed was a period. Karen and Tony had a second son without any problems.

Treatment plans for excesses

BLOOD STASIS

Blood stasis is one of the most common causes of infertility and is commonly associated with patients who have a history of:

- Previous surgical procedures
- Endometriosis
- Polycystic ovaries or PCOS
- Ovarian cysts
- Amenorrhea
- Problems associated with the fallopian tubes, miscarriage and ectopic pregnancy

Signs and symptoms include:

Painful, irregular or late periods, amenorrhea (no periods), scant or profuse bleeding, spotting or interrupted menstruation, dark clotted blood, stabbing localized pain which is worse with pressure and relieved after the discharge of clots, cold limbs, varicose or blue veins on the lower abdomen, haemorrhoids, varicose veins on the legs, and periodic pins and needles or numbness in the limbs. The BBT does not drop on Day 1 of the cycle but temperature remains elevated.

The tongue has a unique role in the diagnosis of Blood stasis. Typically it will look crimson and have purplish spots; the veins under the tongue will be prominent and purplish-blue. This colouration is the result of poor blood circulation, which results in the blood cells being less oxygenated.

The pulse is typically choppy.

What this means

The factors that lead to the development of Blood stasis vary, so it is important to find the cause. A surgical procedure, childbirth, miscarriage or an evacuation of retained products of conception (ERPC) after a miscarriage will traumatize the body, causing normal Blood flow to be interrupted. Any of these can easily lead to stasis if aftercare is not sufficient. An ectopic pregnancy may also be related to Blood stasis.

Conception: Blood stasis will always impede conception because stagnation causes obstruction and prevents normal Blood flow to the reproductive system, particularly to the uterus. This in turn affects the normal functioning of the Conception and Penetrating Vessels (see pages 51–52).

Menstruation: Blood stasis inhibits Blood flow, so menstrual periods may become scant, delayed, irregular (with spotting) or stop altogether (amenorrhea). On the other hand, menstruation may become profuse if the Blood is unable to enter the meridians, thus flow becomes irregular.

Blood stasis can also sometimes cause the Blood to thicken and therefore the menstrual discharge will be dark, contain blood clots and there will be pain when passing clots during menstruation. The pain is experienced as localized stabbing and typically worsens with pressure and is relieved after the discharge of clots.

Ovulation: Blood stasis is a very important consideration when ovulation approaches because the Penetrating Vessel (see pages 51–52) must be full of Blood; or in Western terms, the uterus lining must be ready to receive the fertilized egg.

It is fundamentally important to establish at the beginning of the treatment whether there are symptoms of Blood stasis, so as to clear the way for the treatment to progress.

Treatment principle
Activating Blood circulation and removing Blood stasis.

Typical acupuncture points and explanation
Qi Hai (CV-6) and **Guan Yuan** (CV-4): encourage *qi* to move the blood and eliminate stagnation in the lower abdomen (where most Blood stasis is found).

Xue Hai (SP-10): is most efficient in treating Blood stasis associated with prolonged menstruation and Blood Heat.

San Yin Jiao (SP-6): harmonizes the Liver and invigorates Blood.

Tai Chong (LV-3): promotes free-flowing Liver *qi* and the flow of *qi* throughout the body, particularly to the genitals.

Leading herbal formula
Tao Hong Si Wu Tang, Four herb decoction with safflower and peach kernel (see page 181).

Lifestyle and diet recommendations
Blood stasis always involves *qi* stagnation, so the foods that benefit *qi* flow will also be beneficial for Blood circulation. This is why the dietary recommendations given here are also beneficial for treating Liver *qi* stagnation. Although diet can only be a small part of the treatment for Blood stasis, it is important not to exacerbate existing Blood stasis problems by eating the wrong foods, because toxicity and fat stored in the Blood will also contribute to the condition. The precise diet plan will depend on the root cause of the pattern. The following tips can be easily incorporated into your lifestyle:

- Choose only easily digestible meals.
- Steaming, stir-frying or roasting vegetables is a beneficial way to retain the nutrients.

- Consume one or two units of red wine per week but be aware that you may have conceived if your health is in good form and that alcohol could be harmful to your baby. (There are nine units in an average bottle of wine).
- Avoid cold, raw foods and chilled or iced drinks as they constrict the circulation of *qi* and Blood.
- Exercise regularly to promote good Blood circulation.
- See page 208 for a list of specific recommended foods.

Case study

Sue, aged 37

PROBLEM:	**trying to conceive for 4½ years**
METHODS TRIED:	**IUI, 3 IVF cycles, FET**
TCM OBJECTIVE:	**to clear the abdomen of Blood stasis**
LENGTH OF TREATMENT:	**4 months for the first pregnancy**
OUTCOME:	**4 children in the long term**

Sue was 37 when she came to see us. She had had three spontaneous pregnancies when she was in her twenties and early thirties. The first was miscarried at ten weeks when the embryo stopped developing; the next two pregnancies both resulted in miscarriage at five weeks.

She was waiting for her family doctor to refer her to the hospital for recurrent miscarriage investigation. In the meantime, I had organized an ovarian reserve hormone test for her, which showed everything to be within normal range. Her periods were regular, and apart from being slightly painful, there was no other obvious abnormality.

TCM assessment and treatment plan
Sue had a normal-looking tongue and the coating was normal; she did not complain of any unpleasant period symptoms and her general health seemed to be reasonably good. However, she complained of cold limbs all the time and her pulses were choppy, which is a typical symptom of Blood stasis. I used this as a starting point.

After four weeks of taking herbs to activate the Blood circulation, Sue began feeling much warmer at night; even feeling slightly hot and thirsty – which showed that she also had slight Heat or *yin* deficiency by nature. Therefore, I added some herbal ingredients to complement the treatment.

Four months further into treatment, Sue's period was late and her temperature had remained constantly high since ovulation. I asked Sue to have a home pregnancy test. During her follow-up consultation, she said she had not done the pregnancy test because she had had a period and was now on Day 10 of her cycle. She was terribly disappointed.

However, her temperature still remained at the same high level as before the bleeding. I still believed there could be a pregnancy. I arranged for Sue to go for a Beta HCG blood test to test her human chorionic gonadotropin levels. She was terribly anxious, so I promised her that I would only call her back for a scan if she was pregnant.

When the blood test confirmed that she really was pregnant, I sent her for an ultrasound scan. At eight weeks and six days, Sue found out that she was not only pregnant, but with twins! There could also have been a third pregnancy but only the gestational sac was present, which meant it would not have been able to develop. The blood that Sue lost was not menstrual blood but may have been a fourth pregnancy. The signs were of a natural multiple pregnancy.

Sue went on to full term and gave birth safely to twins: a boy and a girl. Multiple pregnancies as a result of TCM treatment are very uncommon, so I asked Sue whether there was any history of twins in the family. She told me that her grandmother was a twin.

EXCESSIVE LIVER *QI* STAGNATION

Liver *qi* stagnation is common and a prevalent cause of infertility in modern society. It is mainly associated with cases of:

- Unexplained infertility
- Hormonal imbalance
- Problems associated with ovulation and menstruation

When the problem goes untreated, Blood can't circulate in the normal way, which may create Blood stasis. This leads to:

- Endometriosis
- Ovarian cysts
- Problems associated with the fallopian tubes, miscarriage and ectopic pregnancy

Disorders of Liver *qi* are a very common cause of gynaecological conditions, particularly if symptoms are present during ovulation or before menstruation.

The Liver Meridian crosses the pelvis and the reproductive organs. Thus Liver *qi* constraint is easily induced by stress or adverse factors due to the nature of the person's physical condition. A person born with a weak Spleen function could have a lower stress threshold than someone with a strong Spleen function. Liver *qi* stagnation can affect the stages of the menstrual cycle that require movement –

such as the expulsion of the egg, the catching of it by the fallopian tube, the passage of the egg down to the uterus and adapting to changes in hormonal levels. Clinical manifestations of Liver *qi* constraint are prominent before the period, because at this point change needs to be negotiated smoothly and may include irritability, breast soreness, bloating or headaches.

Signs and symptoms include:

A feeling of pressure or a sensation of tightness in the chest or ribs, bloating, cramping or colic pain in the abdomen and upper abdomen, disharmony of the bowel with either constipation and/or diarrhoea, frequent sighing, lateral headaches (headache before or near the start of a period), premenstrual tension with breast distension, irregular menstruation, small blood clots, lack of motivation, cold hands and feet, the feeling of a lump or phlegm in the throat, a sense of frustration or periods of depression and unexplained infertility. The physical and psychological symptoms come and go.

The tongue can be normal red, or pink with a thin coating.

The pulse is wiry and feels taut like a violin string as a result of tension.

What this means

Liver *qi* stagnation is characterized by a feeling of pressure. This results from a blocked flow of *qi*, most commonly caused by long-term emotional strain. The symptoms manifest in different areas depending on the individual (as listed in Signs and symptoms, above). Sighing typically helps to release stagnant *qi* from the chest.

Headaches are caused by stagnant *qi* along the Liver Meridian, and there may be the feeling of a lump or phlegm in the throat as the Liver Meridian passes by there. On an emotional level, restricted *qi* flow leads to a sense of frustration or periods of depression.

Menstruation: Liver *qi* is responsible for free-flowing energy and the movement of Blood; it has an important influence on menstruation, especially in the premenstrual phase. If Liver *qi* stagnates, it causes premenstrual tension with breast distension (where the Liver Meridian also flows), irregular menstruation and small blood clots.

Ovulation: As ovulation involves movement and change, it is important that *qi* flow is free of obstruction during this time. Liver *qi* stagnation can obstruct ovulation. When BBT is erratic in the follicular phase it may be an indication that Liver *qi* is not running smoothly.

In men: Liver *qi* stagnation can result in sperm cells being unable to move correctly. Obstructed *qi* and Blood flow in the groin area and the limbs leads to cold hands and feet.

Typically with *qi* stagnation, physical and psychological symptoms will appear and disappear according to the fluctuation of *qi* flow. Thus physical movement usually improves symptoms while emotional pressure worsens them.

Patients with infertility caused by Liver *qi* stagnation are often classified as having 'unexplained infertility' by medical specialists as *qi* is not recognized in Western medicine.

Note: In some people, Liver *qi* stagnation can easily transform or develop into Liver Heat. So as well as the symptoms listed above, patients often also complain of a sense of pressure on the chest or upper abdomen, irritability, a propensity to outbursts of anger, acid reflux, feeling hot or thirsty with a desire to drink a lot of cold liquids, constipation, difficulty in falling asleep and a slightly rapid pulse.

A WORD ABOUT PERSONALITY

Certain personalities are more prone to Liver *qi* stagnation, particularly sensitive and artistic types. Those who are very creative and are born with a highly sensitive nature are also very delicate mentally and easily take in too much on an emotional level. If you are troubled by insomnia or a disrupted sleep pattern, try the following self-help tips:

- Try to speak and walk more slowly than you usually do. This will avoid unnecessary tension.
- Plan trips and appointments to allow for extra time. It is much better to arrive at your destination early than worry that you might be late due to traffic or any unexpected interruption during the journey.
- Regular exercise is necessary to improve blood circulation and to increase the supply of oxygen to your brain. Swimming, meditation, yoga and Pilates are particularly recommended if you find your sleep pattern has been affected.

Treatment principle
Soothing the Liver and moving *qi*.

Typical acupuncture points and explanation
Tai Chong (LV-3) and **Jie Xi** (ST-41): to free the flow of Liver *qi*.

Qi Hai (CV-6): promotes energy and moves *qi* from the lower abdomen.

Guan Yuan (CV-4): strengthens and supports the movement of *qi* to the uterus.

San Yin Jiao (SP-6): spreads Liver *qi* and nourishes Liver Blood, thus harmonizing the liver.

Yin Tang (EX-HN 3): has a calming function (see illustration, page 232).

Ge Shu (UB-17): is cooling and moves Blood; **Gan Shu** (UB-18): soothes Liver *qi* and regulates the Blood; **Shen Shu** (UB-23): tonifies Kidney *yin* or *yang*.

Leading herbal formula

Xiao Yao Tang, Easy wanderer tea (see page 174–175).

Lifestyle and diet recommendations

Emotions have the greatest influence on the movement of *qi*; however, a balanced diet and healthy lifestyle can support the Liver by promoting the production and flow of *qi* and Blood. Try the following tips:

- Try choosing easily digestible meals, and eating less overall, especially in the evening.
- Eat plenty of fresh fruits, vegetables and salads.
- Grains like barley, rye and rice are beneficial, but only in small amounts.
- Small amounts of mildly bitter foods and spices such as rosemary, coriander or marjoram stimulate Liver *qi*.
- Avoid eating when you are upset.
- Avoid rich and fatty foods, highly processed foods and foods with chemical additives, all of which can obstruct digestion and the flow of *qi*.
- Steaming and stir-frying are the preferred cooking methods.

For Liver *qi* stagnation and excessive Heat

The dietary tips given for Liver *qi* stagnation are also beneficial here, but bear in mind the following tips too:

- Avoid warm, acrid flavours such as chilli and curry.
- Avoid spicy, oily, fatty and deep-fried foods, as these can promote further Heat.
- Foods with a bitter, cool and slightly sour flavour are beneficial.
- See page 209 for a list of specific recommended foods.

Case study

Jacquie, aged 35

PROBLEM:	**symptoms of premature menopause**
METHODS TRIED:	**natural conception**
TCM OBJECTIVE:	**to clear severe Liver *qi* stagnation**
LENGTH OF TREATMENT:	**6 months**
OUTCOME:	**natural conception; a son**

Jacquie was 35 years old when she came to see us. She had been on the contraceptive pill since the age of 29. When she came off the pill, her periods did not return. Her family doctor had arranged some ovarian reserve tests for her which showed that her FSH was 81.8 IU/L, LH was 26 IU/L and oestradiol was low at 56 pmol/L. Repeated tests showed similar results. Her Anti-Mullerian hormone test was less than 0.7 pmol/L.

TCM assessment and treatment plan

She was slimly built, had suffered from high blood pressure for two years and also from hot flushes. Her periods had been regular before she went on the pill, but since the age of 33 she had had only two. The first was 15 days after she came off the pill and the other was two months before coming to see me. She found it difficult to get off to sleep, she felt thirsty and had frequent hot flushes; she felt palpitations often and vibrations on her feet. She had a normal tongue with a cracked texture and a dry and light–normal coating. Her pulses were wiry and rapid.

Jacquie was suffering from severe Liver *qi* stagnation, which had transformed into Heat. It had resulted in amenorrhea and menopausal symptoms. We felt that it would be necessary to help her to clear her excessive Liver Heat and remove the Blood stagnation to help regulate her periods. Only once we were able to get her periods restarted would we be able to try to help her to achieve a more regular cycle, before helping her to conceive again.

During the TCM treatment her general health improved, her sleeping became better and she experienced fewer hot flushes. Her first period returned after four months of TCM treatment.

Her initial cycle was a short one of only 18 days; the next was 35 days. We repeated her hormone test and found her FSH had come down to 5.8 IU/L, oestradiol was very high, but her Anti-Mullerian hormone test had slightly increased to 1.5 pmol/L. We were planning to repeat her hormone test again at a later date but then she discovered she was pregnant. She had a wonderful pregnancy and gave birth to a healthy boy.

EXCESSIVE PHLEGM-DAMP

Phlegm-Damp is one of the most common causes of infertility, mostly linked with female patients who have:

- Polycystic ovaries or PCOS
- Endometriosis
- Problems associated with the fallopian tubes and miscarriage

In men, symptoms include prostate disorders and erectile dysfunction.

Signs and symptoms include:

Delayed menstruation or amenorrhea, obesity or difficulty in losing weight, heavy, sticky or muddy vaginal discharge, mucus in the blood or stool, sticky stools, a pale complexion, urinary difficulties, a feeling of heaviness, difficulty in getting up in the morning, tiredness, needing a lot of sleep or sleeping heavily, phlegm in the throat, a dazed mind or heavy head, oily skin, swelling, oedema, ovarian cyst formation and obstruction or blockage of the fallopian tubes.

The tongue has a characteristically greasy coating.

The pulse is slippery or soggy.

Note: Patients who are diagnosed with polycystic ovaries or PCOS, and are undergoing an assisted fertility procedure, normally respond well to a follicle stimulating hormone injection. These patients' ovaries are like a sponge – puffy and slightly larger than normal, which is due to fluid retention in the ovary. The ovaries also contain a lot of follicles. Sadly, most of the follicles are immature and the quality of the eggs tends to be poor.

What this means

Phlegm-Damp is characterized by stickiness, which is reflected in discharge – for example, greasy sweat. Because Dampness is naturally heavy, it sinks downwards in the body, with symptoms typically occurring in the middle and lower areas.

Dampness: Damp obstruction can cause delayed menstruation or even amenorrhea, muddy vaginal discharge or mucus in the menstrual blood.

In the intestine, Dampness interferes with fluid absorption and stool formation, causing loose sticky stools. There may also be mucus in the stool.

In the bladder, Damp obstruction will cause urinary difficulties and cloudy urine. The heavy nature of Dampness causes a sensation of being weighed down and a feeling of heaviness. Patients with this pattern often find it difficult to get up in the morning, or feel tired throughout the day, but feel better and have more energy as the day goes on.

Phlegm: Phlegm shows up as obstructions in the middle and upper parts of the body. For example, phlegm in the throat area and a dazed mind or heavy head.

Phlegm-Damp can cause a feeling of nausea because it obstructs the digestive system. When Phlegm-Damp accumulates in the skin or muscle tissues it gives rise to oily skin, swelling, oedema, obesity or cyst formation.

In women this pattern can manifest with vaginal discharge, obstructed and prolonged menstrual cycles, fluids blocking the fallopian tubes or the formation of ovarian cysts. In men there may be prostate disorders or erectile dysfunction.

Treatment principle

Eliminating Dampness and resolving obstruction in the lower *jiao* (abdomen).

Typical acupuncture points and explanation

Qi Hai (CV-6) and **Guan Yuan** (CV-4): lift the vital energy, eliminate Dampness and strengthen the uterus.

Yin Ling Quan (SP-9) and **San Yin Jiao** (SP-6): are used to eliminate Dampness and regulate *qi*.

Zu San Li (ST-36): tonifies stomach energy and supports the digestive system.

Feng Long (ST-40): clears phlegm.

Pi Shu (UB-20): improves Spleen *qi*; **Shen Shu** (UB-23): tonifies Kidney *yin* or *yang*; **Dachang Shu** (UB-25): expels excessive Damp and Heat.

Leading herbal formula

Qi Gong San, Arousing the uterus (see page 182).

Lifestyle and diet recommendations

Phlegm-Damp is best prevented by avoiding rich, greasy foods and instead incorporating foods that support fluid transformation and resolve stagnation. Follow these tips:

- Easily digested, simple and cooked foods are beneficial as they support the Spleen *qi* to transform Dampness and Phlegm.
- Add healthy spices to your meals.
- Barley, wholegrain rice, buckwheat and oats are beneficial when consumed in small quantities.
- Avoid fatty meats like duck, goose, sausages or deep-fried foods.
- Avoid sweets, sugar, dairy products like milk, cheese, cream and butter, fizzy drinks, chocolate and cloying foods like avocados, bananas and pears.
- Exercise regularly to promote energy.
- Have small, frequent meals to improve the metabolism.
- Avoid drinking alcohol.
- See pages 209–210 for a list of specific recommended foods.

Case study

Maggie, 32

PROBLEM:	**severe endometriosis and PCOS**
METHODS TRIED:	**natural conception**
TCM OBJECTIVE:	**to clear Phlegm-Damp in the abdomen and the uterus**
LENGTH OF TREATMENT:	**5 months for the first pregnancy**
OUTCOME:	**natural conception; 3 children in the long term**

Maggie was 32 and her husband was 33 years old. They had tried to conceive for over two years but had never achieved a pregnancy. She was overweight, which may have been due to her body carrying too much Phlegm and Damp. Her cycles were between 22 and 28 days with a five-day bleed. She complained that the bleeding was slightly heavy, the colour was mainly dark brown and she suffered from slightly painful periods. Her husband's semen analysis was normal.

TCM assessment and treatment plan

A laparoscopy revealed severe endometriosis and PCOS. Following laser treatment for endometriosis on the back of the uterus, the patency of her fallopian tubes was confirmed. She received TCM treatment for five months before conceiving successfully and giving birth to her first child. Subsequently she conceived again without any help from us and the couple now have three children.

EXCESSIVE DAMP-HEAT

Damp-Heat is another common cause of infertility, and is prevalent in my fertility clinic. The problem is associated mainly with patients who have a history of:

- Pelvic Inflammatory Disease (PID)
- Chlamydia
- Recurrent cystitis or urinary tract infections
- Endometriosis
- Problems associated with the fallopian tubes, miscarriage and ectopic pregnancy

Men will often have itchiness or spots in the groin area, cloudy urine, a low sperm count, low sperm motility or a high number of abnormal sperm.

Signs and symptoms include:

Irregular menstrual bleeding including postmenstrual or premenstrual spotting, lower abdominal pain with heaviness, abdominal distension and bloated stomach, nausea, puffy hands and feet, lower backache, greasy, yellow sweat, genital herpes, sweating and itching in the genital area, vaginal itching, yellow and unpleasant-smelling discharge, inflammation in the vagina and urethra in women or in the penis in men, loose stools with a fetid odour, a burning sensation in the anus and dark urine or frequent urination.

The tongue is greasy with a coating turned yellow by the Heat.

The pulse might be rapid, representing the Heat; and slippery or soggy, showing Damp.

What this means
No one is born with Damp and Heat in the body. Damp-Heat symptoms often develop when the abdominal area has become inflamed, or following a surgical procedure in which the abdominal environment has been traumatized; or where there is underlying infection. They can also be caused by a malfunction of the digestive system, where fluids are under constant attack from an unhealthy diet that includes heavy alcohol intake, too much curry and chilli, or too many iced or chilled drinks. If stomach fluids have to overwork, digestion slows down and excess fluid overloads the lower part of body; therefore, the lower abdomen feels heavy. The Heat will also cause puffy hands and feet.

Menstruation: When symptoms of Heat and Damp combine and obstruct the lower part of the abdomen it could lead to the development of Blood stasis. This is characterized by painful periods, constant abdominal discomfort or pain, yellowish sticky discharge or itching. The combination of Damp and Heat causes light sweating throughout the day (steaming). Typically the sweat is greasy and yellow, which tends to stain clothes.

Treatment principle
Eliminating Dampness, clearing Heat from the lower abdomen and activating the flow of Blood.

Typical acupuncture points and explanation
Guan Yuan (CV-4) and **Zhong Ji** (CV-3): used together to regulate and strengthen the uterus, and to remove Damp-Heat obstruction from the genital system.

Yin Ling Quan (SP-9) and **San Yin Jiao** (SP-6): to eliminate Dampness and regulate *qi*.

Feng Long (ST-40): to eliminate Phlegm-Damp.

Leading herbal formulas
Xue Fu Zhu Yu Tang, Drive out stasis in the middle and lower abdomen tea (see pages 173–174).

Bi Xie Fen Qing Tang, Draining Dampness tea (see pages 180–181).

Lifestyle and diet recommendations

Damp and Heat upset the lower part of the body, which is closely related to the digestive system, so foods that benefit digestion and reactivate Blood flow will be important. Try these self-help tips:

- Eat only foods that are easily digestible.
- Foods that are particularly beneficial include grains such as barley and rye, soda bread and root vegetables.
- Steaming, stir-frying or roasting vegetables is a beneficial way to retain nutrients.
- Avoid drinking alcohol.
- Avoid foods that are oily, deep-fried, fatty or spicy. Avoid curries.
- Avoid cold, raw foods and chilled or iced drinks as they constrict the circulation of *qi* and Blood.
- Exercise regularly to promote good Blood circulation.
- See page 210 for a list of specific recommended foods.

Case study

Jared, aged 26

PROBLEM: **male infertility**

METHODS TRIED: **natural conception**

TCM OBJECTIVE: **to clear excessive Damp and Heat**

LENGTH OF TREATMENT: **1st child 3½ months, 2nd child 6 months**

OUTCOME: **natural conception; 2 children in the long term**

Jared had only one testicle. The other had been removed when he was a child following an unsuccessful operation to aid testicular descent. He had a low sperm count and was able to produced only 5 million sperm in his entire semen sample. He was concerned that there was a causal link between the two.

Jared had a disturbed sleep pattern, woke up frequently, feeling hot and sweaty, and had vivid dreams. He also had frequent and loose bowel movements, three to four times a day, and complained that his urine was dark with an unpleasant smell. He often felt thirsty. He had a normal, light-coloured tongue, with a thick and yellow coating. His pulse was aggressively slippery and rapid. Jared's symptoms were typical signs of excessive Damp and Heat.

TCM assessment

Having a single testicle does not necessarily result in a low sperm count as the remaining testicle should still be able to function normally and produce enough sperm for conception. There was a possibility that physical trauma caused by the surgery might have had an indirect impact on the abdominal environment. It was also possible that Jared's unhealthy diet was having an effect. His alcohol intake was low (he drank the equivalent of only one or two units per week) but he was slightly overweight and enjoyed chilled drinks straight from the fridge, as well as spicy curries and chilli, all of which can inflame the abdominal environment.

Frequent and loose bowels and dark-smelling urine may be signs that unhealthy digestive fluids are building up and obstructing the lower abdomen. This restricts the movement of fluids and healthy circulation in the body.

TCM treatment plan

The aim was to clear Jared's abdominal obstruction and reduce the Heat. After only two weeks of herbal medication, Jared found that his urine was much clearer than before and the frequency of his bowel movements had reduced to two to three times a day. He was sleeping better and dreaming less, and he felt more energetic. He felt generally much less hot and sweaty.

By the second month of his TCM treatment, Jared's semen sample had improved dramatically, increasing from 5 million in the total semen sample to 19.6 million per ml. His previous semen sample had been so poor that it was impossible to carry out a motility test. This time the situation was quite different.

A further six weeks of TCM treatment followed, with no changes to the herbal medication. His sperm count decreased during this period to 6.1 million per ml. However, he was now showing the best sperm motility rate to date, and the rate of forward progression was also much improved. These factors are more important than high sperm count alone. Jared reported at this point that his wife had become pregnant.

One and a half years after the birth of their first baby, Jared returned to see us again to attempt a second pregnancy. I urged Jared to consider bringing his wife to see me as I thought that her fertility potential may have dropped following the birth of her first baby. I knew I could help his wife to improve the health of her reproductive system, which would also help to overcome the effect of Jared's low sperm count. IVF could also be considered as his sample would be good enough for an ICSI cycle.

The couple were still young and there was no reason why they should not continue to try to conceive in the way they had chosen, for a longer time. However, Jared put my mind at rest and promised to bring his wife to see me should no pregnancy be achieved in the next few months. Happily, after six months of TCM treatment (double the treatment time taken for their first baby), Jared's wife conceived again and went full term before giving birth to their second healthy baby.

Note: This was not the first case where I have seen a male's semen quantity and quality drop once TCM treatment ends. No matter what we did for Jared, his sperm count did not increase as much as we expected. However, I believe the TCM treatment will have reduced the level of chromosome abnormality, which would not show under normal semen analysis.

EXCESSIVE BLOOD HEAT

Excessive Heat in the Blood is not unusual in cases of infertility. It is most often associated with patients who show signs of:

- Peri-menopausal symptoms with short menstrual cycles
- Raised FSH levels
- A poor response to IVF stimulation (see below)

Signs and symptoms include:

A short menstrual cycle, heavy bleeding during menstruation, pain during menstruation, dark or bright red menstrual blood, a feeling of heat, thirst, skin rashes, constipation, yellow urine, aversion to heat, anxiety, mental restlessness, poor egg quality and a thin endometrium. Patients also exhibit a poor response to FSH during IVF: either the follicles grow very fast and very big but there is no egg inside, or ovulation takes place before egg collection.

The tongue is red and has a slim body.

The pulse is rapid and fine.

What this means

The symptoms and signs of Heat in the Blood depend on the organ involved. For example, in TCM the Heart is the house of the mind, so if Heart Blood has Heat it agitates the mind, causing anxiety and mental restlessness.

When Blood Heat affects the womb and Penetrating Vessel (see pages 51–52), the Heat causes the Blood to 'overflow' from the vessel. This results in heavy and premature bleeding, and typically also a feeling of heat in the genital region during menstruation. Generally, Heat is not conducive to the development of good-quality eggs or a healthy womb lining, so it hampers fertilization and implantation.

Blood Heat in the intestines or bladder will dry the stool and urine, causing constipation or yellow urine and there may even be blood in the stool or urine. When Liver Blood has Heat it is characterized by red and itching skin rashes. Heat in the Blood accelerates the Blood flow and empties fluids, hence the pulse will be rapid or fine.

Treatment principle

Clearing Heat, cooling the Blood and regulating menstruation.

Typical acupuncture points and explanation

Xue Hai (SP-10) and *Ge Shu* (UB-17): clear Heat and cool the Blood.

Tai Chong (LV-3): reduce Liver Heat downwards; regulate Blood and the gynaecological system.

Tai Xi (KID-3) and *Zhao Hai* (KID-6): cool the Blood, nourish *yin* and regulate the Blood and genitals.

Qu Chi (LI-11) and *He Ku* (LI-4): allow the Heat to expel from the outer body.

Leading herbal formula

Qing Jing Tang, Clear the menses formula (see page 184).

Lifestyle and diet recommendations

- Avoid spicy, hot and drying foods like curry, pepper, ginger, garlic and cinnamon.
- Cooling foods are of great benefit, such as melon, banana, watermelon, cucumber, celery and lettuce.
- Try to eat lots of fresh fruit and vegetables.
- Eat a light breakfast.
- Reduce alcohol intake.
- Take light exercise.
- See page 210–211 for a list of specific recommended foods.

Case study

Ali, aged 32

PROBLEM:	**no periods for 2 years**
METHODS TRIED:	**natural conception**
TCM OBJECTIVE:	**to clear Blood Heat**
LENGTH OF TREATMENT:	**4 months**
OUTCOME:	**natural conception; a daughter**

Ali and her husband, Martin, were one of the most anxious couples I have ever treated as Ali had been diagnosed with early menopause. They came to see me when Ali was 32. She had had an abortion when she was 29 following an unplanned pregnancy; she then went on the pill for two years. Since coming off the pill, she had had no periods at all for two years. She was desperately upset.

TCM assessment and treatment plan

Ali's FSH level was alarmingly high, measuring 69, then 82: a level more typical of someone in their post-menopausal years. She had other typical menopausal symptoms too: powerful, aggressive pulse, Heat and a red tongue. Internally, there was clearly a lot of emotion boiling away. I was unable to promise Ali anything, but I knew that I needed to clear some of the Heat and get her Blood flowing healthily again; then we could see whether we might get her periods starting again.

After three months of TCM treatment, Ali had her first period and her FSH level dropped down to 10. However, her oestrogen levels were very high, which may have suppressed her FSH level. She had another ovulation cycle after 40 days and I was unable to repeat her FSH and oestrogen level tests again – but she conceived naturally, straight away. The relief for the couple was huge and helped Ali to deal with a lot of unresolved emotion concerning the abortion that had been stirring within her.

COLD IN THE UTERUS

Cold in the uterus (womb) affects the health of a pregnancy. Either the woman finds it difficult to conceive or may experience complications during pregnancy. This condition is associated mainly with:

- A history of miscarriage
- A history of stillbirth
- Polycystic ovaries or PCOS
- Uterine fibroids

Signs and symptoms include:

Late or absent periods, cramping pain during periods, dark menstrual blood with clots, brown spotting before a period, periods that stop and start, a dislike of cold, a general feeling of cold or a feeling of cold from the waist down as if sitting in cold water, shivering, white vaginal discharge and lumps or masses in the uterus.

The tongue is bluish-purple or pale with a wet coating.

The pulse may be full and tight (excess Cold) or weak (deficient Cold).

What this means

Cold invades, constricts and slows down Blood flow, causing Blood stasis in the meridians and in the uterus. Blood stasis causes the Blood to thicken, which results in poor Blood circulation, causing the veins to appear blue because the blood cells are less oxygenated.

Menstrual flow will not be smooth, there may be dark clotted blood and a feeling of cold. Menstrual pain will be typically relieved by warmth because the warmth temporarily aids the flow of Blood. External Cold often combines with external Dampness to exacerbate Blood stasis. In severe cases, Blood stasis may form lumps or masses in the abdomen, causing a feeling of heat.

Excess Cold patterns generally last only a short time, because after a prolonged period excessive Cold will lead to a deficiency of *yang* instead. The clinical manifestations of both patterns are similar because they are of the same nature.

Excess Cold: the signs and symptoms have an acute onset, the pain is more severe, the pulse is full and tight and the tongue has a thick white coating. The condition does not last a long time.

Deficient Cold: the signs and symptoms will reflect the lack of *qi* to warm the body because it is a result of deficiency. Hence menstrual pain is dull and the menstrual period will be weak. With this pattern, the deficient *yang* is too weak to move the Blood, thereby causing Blood stasis, manifesting with dark clots. The deficiency of *yang* will be too weak to warm the body, causing shivering and an aversion to cold.

Treatment principle
Dispelling Cold, eliminating Blood stasis and warming the uterus.

Typical acupuncture points and explanation
Qi Hai (CV-6) and **Guan Yuan** (CV-4): are used with moxa on the needle to warm Kidney *yang*, expel Cold and strengthen the uterus.

San Yin Jiao (SP-6): reinforces *yang* and has a warming function.

Zhao Hai (KID-6): regulates the lower *jiao*, benefits the Kidney and relieves pain.

Leading herbal formula
Gui Zhi Fu Ling Tang, Cinnamon twig and poria decoction (see page 183).

Lifestyle and diet recommendations
A diet that boosts *yang* and promotes Blood circulation will supplement TCM treatment to warm the uterus, expel Cold and remove stasis.

- Roasted meats and warming stews are recommended.
- Avoid cold drinks and raw food.
- Increase exercise levels, but make sure you warm up first.
- See page 211 for a list of specific recommended foods.

COLD IN THE UTERUS AND KIDNEY *YANG* DEFICIENCY
Cold in the uterus rarely occurs on its own. It is more usually associated with Kidney *yang* deficiency.

Treatment plans for deficiencies

BLOOD AND *QI* DEFICIENCY

In TCM, a woman's physiology is determined by Blood whereas in men it is determined by *qi*. Therefore women and men with Blood and *qi* deficiency typically present with:

- Infertility with low oestradial (see box, 156) production
- Poor response to IVF stimulation
- Poor fertilization
- Prolonged menstruation
- Polycystic ovaries or PCOS
- Amenorrhea
- Low libido

Men may present with low sperm motility, low libido and/or erection problems.

Often problems will have developed after illness or surgical intervention or as the result of a weak constitution.

Signs and symptoms include:

Dry skin, brittle nails, lustreless dull hair, anxiety, neurosis, disturbed sleep, palpitations, light dizziness, headaches that become worse when tired or during periods, delayed menstruation, light and scant menstrual bleeding with pale pink or watery and brownish blood, abdominal pain or headaches after periods, poor appetite, pale complexion, decreased libido and difficulty achieving an erection and weakness.

The tongue is light pink and paler than a normal tongue.

The pulse is fine and deep. There is a lack of strength in the pulse.

What this means

The function of Blood in TCM is to nurture and moisten the body. In TCM, 'Blood deficiency' does not mean a *lack* of Blood but a lack of *nourishing* Blood. Low Blood nourishment will affect all aspects of the body, and this is the cause of dry skin, brittle nails, lustreless dull hair, pale complexion and pale tongue.

Fertility: Blood deficiency can lead to insufficient nourishment of the foetus and of the mucus membranes of the uterus. Hence the endometrium will be thin and not conducive to effective implantation, and the foetus may not be nourished adequately.

If accompanying *qi* deficiency occurs, the foetus may not grow and thrive adequately, or the uterus may not be strong enough to hold the foetus. This often causes problems after about 14 to 15 weeks of pregnancy when the foetus is starting to grow larger.

The mind: Blood also nourishes the mind. When Blood (and *qi*) are deficient, the mind is unbalanced; hence there will be uneasiness, anxiety, neurosis and disturbed sleep. Because Blood contains *qi*, a deficiency of one will also affect the other (for example, when Heart *qi* becomes deficient there will be palpitations because there is not enough *qi* to move the Blood supply to the Heart). Blood becomes more deficient when a person is tired or during menstruation so dizziness and light headaches may be worse at these times.

In women: Blood deficiency affects women more than men. Women with this pattern may have insufficient Blood in a regular 28-day cycle to fill the Penetrating Vessel (see pages 51–52) and uterus for menstruation. Therefore the menstrual period is delayed, starting after 32 days or even later. When Liver Blood is deficient, the uterus is supplied with an insufficient amount of Blood, causing light and scant menstrual bleeding, which is pale pink or watery and brownish in colour. Menstrual pain occurs after a period because it is a deficient pattern. Patients with this pattern tend to have low levels of oestradiol in the blood.

In men: Male orgasms depend primarily on *qi* as does the rapid movement of sperm. Hence men with *qi* deficiency may experience a decreased libido, difficulty achieving an erection and overall weakness. There may also be seminal emission without sexual activity.

WHAT IS OESTRADIOL?

Oestradiol is the most important form of oestrogen and is responsible for follicle development during a woman's fertile years. It is produced and released from the ovaries, adrenal cortex and the placenta. Oestradiol is also responsible for the growth of the uterus, fallopian tubes and vagina, as well as promoting breast development and the growth of the outer genitals. It plays a critical role in bone development and in reproductive and sexual functioning. It also influences the metabolism of female body fat and its distribution.

Treatment principle
Nourishing Blood and *qi*.

Typical acupuncture points and explanation
Qi Hai (CV-6) and **Guan Yuan** (CV-4): nourish Blood and *qi* and strengthen the uterus.

Zu San Li (ST-36) and **San Yin Jiao** (SP-6): nourish Blood.

Ge Shu (UB-17) and **Shen Shu** (UB-23): nourish Blood and strengthen the Kidney.

Leading herbal formula

Tiao Jing Tang, Regulate the period tea (see page 177–178).

Lifestyle and diet recommendations

Moistening and nourishing foods that supplement *yin* will also be beneficial for supplementing the Blood. Try the following self-help tips:

- Eat plenty of dark green vegetables rich in chlorophyll, such as spinach, broccoli and green beans.
- Include lots of protein-rich foods in your diet – liver, squid and oysters are especially beneficial.
- Grains, such as oats and rice, can have a nourishing effect.
- The foods listed on pages 212–213, which supplement *yin*, are also useful for treating this pattern.
- Try to steam, roast or blanch foods rather than frying or grilling.
- Avoid spices that dry fluids and Blood, like curry spices and chilli.
- See pages 211–212 for a list of specific recommended foods.

Case study

Terri, aged 27

PROBLEM:	**underweight; no periods for 2 years**
METHODS TRIED:	**natural conception**
TCM OBJECTIVE:	**to regenerate *qi* levels**
LENGTH OF TREATMENT:	**6 months**
OUTCOME:	**natural conception; a son**

Terri and Lucas came to see me even though Terri was very young, just 27. She'd had no periods for two years and was very underweight. They had spent much of that time travelling around the world. She said she felt well and lived a very healthy lifestyle, but admitted she was tired a lot of the time.

TCM assessment and treatment plan

Terri ate lots of fresh fruit and nuts – and very little else – and went running every evening. Lucas's sperm count was perfectly normal and his motility levels were good so I concentrated on persuading Terri to change her lifestyle and build up her energy reserves. I asked her not to go running more than twice a week, and put her on a programme of eating regular meals, three times a day. I told her to have protein at breakfast and fruit snacks in between meals.

I also treated Terri's digestive system with TCM herbs to make sure that she was absorbing all the nutrients and metabolizing her food properly to build up her *qi*. Sure enough, once she started to nourish her body properly, with enough time to rest and regenerate her *qi* levels, her periods restarted – within a couple of months. They now have a healthy son. Terri balances her lifestyle better now. You can't run a body on an empty fuel tank.

KIDNEY *YIN* DEFICIENCY

Kidney *yin* is the basic material for the essence (see page 23), which produces bone marrow and plays a fundamental role in fertility.

Yin enables the egg to ripen and mucus to become fertile. It increases the blood supply to the endometrium so that it thickens. Kidney *yin* can be overused or damaged by lifestyle factors such as overwork, poor diet or inadequate sleep. Kidney *yin* deficiency shows up in the presence of symptoms such as a lack of fertile mucus, a dry vagina or sore vulva during intercourse, infrequent or no periods. In addition, *yin* deficiency can give rise to Heat, which in turn will exacerbate the *yin* deficiency and dry the Blood. This is seen in cases of severe amenorrhea (lack of periods) where the *yin* and the Blood are depleted with accompanying Heat symptoms such as night sweats and dry mouth.

During the peri-menopause and menopause, Kidney *yin* deficiency causes essence to diminish. Symptoms often appear in the area of the lower spinal column and the lower extremities, taking the form of lower back pain or weak knees. Premature ejaculation may develop in men and there may be low ovarian reserve and light or irregular menstrual cycles in women. There may also be a link with the onset of osteoporosis. In TCM, the functioning of the Kidney is also linked to the ears so Kidney *yin* deficiency may also manifest as impaired hearing or tinnitus.

In TCM there is a lot of focus on older women having Kidney *yin* deficiency (see box, opposite), but there are also many younger women whose ovaries have aged prematurely who may also suffer from this condition. This can be due to their natural constitution (at birth), or other medical conditions such as previous illness or surgery. The reproductive organs may be affected and unable to function fully without assistance.

Kidney *yin* deficiency is often associated with:

- Anovulation (a menstrual cycle where no egg is produced or the follicle is under-developed)
- Luteal phase defect
- Immunological infertility (see page 105)

- Low ovarian reserve (showing as a poor response during IVF stimulation; when follicles develop too slowly or too fast; or when there are many immature follicles but not enough mature eggs develop)
- Fluctuating FSH and/or low Anti-Mullerian hormone levels

Men with Kidney *yin* deficiency may suffer from poor sperm production.

KIDNEY *YIN* DEFICIENCY, AGE AND PREGNANCY

As we have seen, the peri-menopause is a ten-year period between the ages of 35 and 45 during which a woman's reproductive capacity begins to decline. Follicle production and egg quality decline as age increases, then end completely during the menopause.

Often women will start to present fluctuating FSH levels and a low Anti-Mullerian hormone level, which shows that the ovaries are vulnerable, malfunctioning or appear to be working harder, and the egg reserve is running low. Once the FSH level is raised and the Anti-Mullerian hormone level is low, a fertility clinic will usually advise women to consider using donor eggs. Can TCM help in a situation like this? The answer is yes...in some cases.

Statistics at our clinic show that *of those who achieve pregnancy*, 29 per cent of women are aged between 40 and 44. (That is not to say that if a woman of 44 turns up to see us she can expect to achieve the same result as patients who began treatment at a younger age. It may take a year or two to achieve a pregnancy.) This compares with 33 per cent of those younger than 35 years old; and a further 33 per cent of those between the ages of 36 and 39, provided they receive the right help and follow our treatment programme.

However, from the age of 45 onwards, the success rate is much reduced and is closer to 5 per cent. Only a handful of women (less than ten) who have conceived with our help at the age of 46 will achieve a live birth. We have also helped women who want to try to become pregnant at the ages of 47, 48 and 50 years old but, sadly, with no live birth.

Note: All of the pregnancies achieved from age 45 onwards were spontaneous pregnancies, or occasionally conceived on a natural cycle IUI. None of them was the result of IVF or ICSI.

Signs and symptoms include:

Dry skin and mucous membranes, dry throat, thirst, constipation, scanty and darkish urination, weight loss, slight dizziness, low-pitched tinnitus, thinning or loss of hair, lower backache, weak knees, loss of teeth, delayed or shortened menstrual periods with scant or watery and bright red blood.

Advanced Kidney *yin* deficiency and its associated Heat show up in the form of hot flushes, night sweats, a feeling of heat that increases in the afternoon, heat sensations on the palms, soles of the feet and centre of the chest, a sense of restlessness, anxiety and insomnia, dry throat at night, scanty darkish urine and dry stools. Occasionally an overactive thyroid may also relate to this pattern.

The tongue has no coating; normal to reddish in colour.

The pulse is fine or weak.

What this means

As Kidney *yin* is seen as the basis material of essence and the 'lower source of water', Kidney *yin* deficiency typically manifests with signs and symptoms of dryness. Hence there will be dry skin and mucous membranes, lack of tongue coating, dry throat, thirst, constipation or scanty and darkish urination. A deficiency in essence (which is related to ageing, see page 158) will weaken the chances of gestation.

It is the function of *yin* to nourish the body and to support the 'structure' of the body. Kidney essence relies on a healthy supply of Kidney *yin* to support the creation of bone marrow and protein in the blood. If the bone marrow is depleted, lower back pain, weak knees and loss of teeth will result. There may also be slight dizziness and low-pitched tinnitus. Kidney health is often reflected in the health of the hair, so Kidney essence or Kidney *yin* deficiency leads to hair thinning or loss.

If Kidney essence is running low, so it cannot produce enough *yin*, this may cause Heat to rise; which can lead to dehydration and therefore fluid loss and weight loss.

Menstruation and ovulation: A deficiency in Kidney *yin* will result in delayed menstrual periods or scant, bright red blood. Prolonged *yin* deficiency may cause Heat in the body to rise and the period of menstruation to be short. This is because there is insufficient nourishment for the follicles to reach maturity; the follicles grow too fast and burst before the egg inside matures. The BBT will reflect this, with an extended follicular phase, longer than the normal 14 days.

Menstrual bleeding is typically light and infrequent, or there will be amenorrhea because there is not enough *yin* to thicken and nourish the endometrium (womb lining). Hence women with *yin* deficiency typically have a thin and poorly nourished endometrium and the embryo may not thrive. An endometrial lining that has not developed soundly may also cause mid-cycle bleeding.

Advanced Kidney *yin* deficiency may further dry up *yin* fluids, causing ascending Heat sensations and flushing of the cheeks. The Heat may also interfere with the functioning of the ovaries. If fertilization does occur, the *yin* deficiency Heat may cause a miscarriage in the early stages of pregnancy, because it can dry the endometrium and force Blood from the vessels supplying the womb. Moreover, many cases of premature menopause are caused by Kidney *yin* deficiency. Patients typically present with night sweats because *yin* dominates at night and the Heat causes *yin* fluids to evaporate. *Yin* essence is lost in the sweat, which further aggravates the *yin* deficiency.

In men: Kidney *yin* deficiency is associated with problems with seminal fluid, sperm count and morphology. *Yin* deficiency Heat is the main cause of azoospermia (low sperm count) because it prevents the sperm from producing cells to function well. The sperm become less able to move efficiently and less able to penetrate the egg.

The quantity and quality of the seminal fluid may also be compromised. The Heat may lead to hyperactivity and increased libido but this is usually accompanied by premature ejaculation and the inability to sustain an erection for long. In addition, the internal Heat may cause inflammation of the prostate gland.

Psychological factors: On a psychological level, patients may feel an internal disquiet or restlessness, and suffer a sense of fear and insomnia, characterized by waking up in the early hours of the morning because the Heat disturbs the mind.

Treatment principle
Nourishing Kidney *yin* and essence.

Typical acupuncture points and explanation
Qi Hai (CV-6) and **Guan Yuan** (CV-4): strengthen the Kidney, nourish Kidney *yin*, regulate the lower *jiao* (abdomen) and strengthen the uterus.

Tai Xi (KID-3), **San Yin Jiao** (SP-6) and **Zhao Hai** (KID-6): nourish Kidney *yin*.

Alternatively:

Ge Shu (UB-17) and **Gan Shu** (UB-18): nourish Liver Blood

Shen Shu (UB-23) and **Tai Xi** (KID-3): tonify Kidney *yin*.

Leading herbal formulas
Liu Wei Di Huang Tang, Six flavour tea (see pages 176–177).

Zhi Bai Di Huang Tang, Eight flavour tea (see page 177). The formula provides a cooling effect when *yin* deficiency Heat is raised.

Bu Yin Jian, Tea to reinforce *yin* (see pages 178–180).

Lifestyle and diet recommendations
A *yin*-supplementing diet follows the same principles as one used for nourishing Blood. Moistening foods and foods that nourish the body stimulate fluid production and therefore supplement *yin* energy. Try to follow these tips:

- Choose neutral protein foods, such as chicken, fish and eggs. Red meats should be eaten only occasionally and in small quantities as they may dry *yin* and Blood.
- Nuts, seeds and soy products are also good protein choices.
- Eat plenty of fresh fruits and vegetables, particularly leafy green vegetables.
- Avoid warming herbs and spices such as cloves, thyme, curry spices, chilli, pepper and cinnamon.
- Try to steam or boil foods, rather than grilling or deep-frying.
- Use fresh stock to make soups (see page 215)
- See pages 212–213 for a list of specific recommended foods.

Case study

Serena, aged 40

PROBLEM:	**endometriosis, peri-menopause**
METHODS TRIED:	**9 ICSI cycles over 10 years**
TCM OBJECTIVE:	**to improve ovarian health**
LENGTH OF TREATMENT:	**30 months**
OUTCOME:	**TCM- and ICSI-assisted conception; twins**

Serena and her husband had been trying to conceive for ten years and had failed nine ICSI cycles before she turned to TCM. She was 40. She had never conceived and had been found to suffer from extensive endometriosis. Following a laparoscopy to clear the endometriosis, she was put on a six-month course of Zoladex (a type of chemical injection that is believed to dry up the endometriosis.) Serena's husband had a very low sperm count: less than 1 million per ml and poor motility of less than 10 per cent.

The couple's nine ICSI cycles had each resulted in a maximum of five follicles being developed. No more than one egg was collected in each cycle; sometimes there were none. Her FSH level was between 11 and 14, which was on the high side of borderline. She had been told that her egg quality was always very poor.

There were several possible reasons for this:

- The results of a post-coital test to examine the interaction between her partner's sperm and the mucus in her cervix suggested that the mucus was hostile to the sperm. (This meant that the sperm could not survive after entering the cervix and it was therefore unable to swim through the cervix to meet the egg.)

- Her husband had an extremely low sperm count.

- She had poor ovarian function: over the years her FSH level had become elevated and was registering at around 13.5 iu/L.

The problems that Serena presented were typical of many of the women who come to see me when assisted fertility treatment has been unsuccessful. She couldn't conceive without intervention and her husband had a severely low sperm count. Even though she was young, she had peri-menopausal symptoms as her ovaries were like those of an older woman. I decided to focus on treating Serena only initially, because men respond more quickly to treatment and a low sperm count can be overcome by using ICSI treatment provided the sperm is healthy.

WHY DOES ENDOMETRIOSIS RETURN?

A laparoscopy is technically effective, but removing the endometriosis does not prevent it from recurring. I always describe the process as being like having leaks in the roof of your house. You may collect all the water, drip by drip, in a series of buckets, but that won't stop the roof leaking again because it doesn't fix the source of the problem.

TCM assessment and treatment plan

Owing to Serena's medical history, I advised the couple to give Serena time to improve her ovary function to benefit egg quality so that the assisted reproduction team would have more mature follicles to work from (and a better chance of fertilization). The consultant was very supportive of her trying TCM and we cooperated well.

I used acupuncture and prescribed various herbal teas, charted her BBT and analysed her pulse and tongue. But no matter which approach I took, I was unable to completely rebalance her system. At the point when her FSH dropped to a good level at 4, her temperature wasn't right; when her FSH changed to borderline high, everything else suddenly looked good.

Serena was desperate to try again and so began a new round of ICSI. Again it was unsuccessful. I advised her to stop the ICSI process and wait until I gave her the go ahead. This time she was ready to give the TCM a chance to work. It took another year, but they had decided that this would be Serena's last round of ICSI and so they were very patient. Eventually, Serena's menstrual cycle became beautifully regular at 26 to 28 days. After three regular cycles and some ovarian reserve tests at the beginning of her cycle, I told Serena she was ready to start ICSI again. Then she developed a cold, which meant she had to stop the TCM. She begged her consultant to let her suspend the cycle and to start again when she was better.

Once well, we began again. Exactly as before, Serena produced only five follicles. But this time, all the follicles grew to a healthy size of 12–14 mm. Five eggs were mature enough to be collected and three were fertilized.

I always explain to patients that the purpose of TCM is to help the ovaries to function more healthily. I could not have used TCM to improve the number of follicles Serena produced, because her cycle showed consistently, over many years, that five was the maximum number her body would manage. By using the herbal treatments and acupuncture I was able to improve her ovary function, which allowed the number of follicles she had available to respond well and to mature to a viable size.

Serena conceived and gave birth to twins: a boy and a girl. She wrote to tell me how proud she was of the children, they looked so gorgeous and healthy. They will be nearly 12 years old by now.

If I was treating Serena and her husband today, I would do something for her husband too. I didn't focus on him initially because she had responded so badly to assisted fertility treatment over so many years that I knew there was a lot of work to be done. I concentrated on Serena in the hope that she might then be able to conceive by herself.

BEWARE OF COLDS

If a patient develops a cold or other illness when they are being treated with TCM, we advise them to stop drinking the teas straight away. This is because the tea works on the main organs of the body at a systemic level. They are very strong and powerful. Sometimes the effect of the tea will take a cold down deeper into the body and it will take longer to clear.

KIDNEY *YANG* DEFICIENCY

Kidney *yang* is responsible for regulating water in the body. It influences the body's metabolism and governs growth, development and reproduction.

Kidney *yang* enhances the vital energy necessary to encourage *yin* and Blood circulation. It encourages egg and sperm production and development, aids sperm motility in men and warms the uterus in women, an important role in fertility – particularly in implantation.

Kidney *yang* deficiency is commonly associated with patients who have a history of:

- Blocked fallopian tubes (fluid in the tubes)
- Anovulation (see page 158)
- Polycystic ovaries or PCOS
- A low progesterone level in the luteal phrase
- Severe endometriosis
- Low seminal fluids and low sperm motility

Signs and symptoms include:

Aversion to cold, cold feet, knees and lower back, low BBT in the luteal phase, a pale, swollen and wet tongue, backache, weakness of the legs and knees, aggravation of symptoms during cold and rainy weather, weakened will, frequent and clear urination, puffiness and oedema especially in the legs, watery discharge, delayed onset of menstruation, scant, light-coloured menstrual blood, loose stools, weakness and lassitude, decreased libido, apathy, increased whitish vaginal discharge, premature greying of head hair, weakness to sustain erection, premature ejaculation or impotence.

Kidney *yang* also controls the pelvic floor, the urinary tract and the reproductive organs. When weakened, there may be night-time incontinence. Men may experience impotence.

The tongue has a pale body.

The pulse is deep and slow.

What this means

Kidney *yin* and Kidney *yang* are intimately interconnected so a deficiency of one will ultimately weaken the other. If Kidney *yang* deficiency is predominant, the following problems may arise.

When Kidney *yang* fails to nourish the Spleen, stools become loose. Muscles also lack nourishment, causing weakness and lassitude. With this pattern, hypothyroidism can develop. As the Kidney constitutes the will, a person with this pattern often has a weakened will and lack of determination.

Cold: Primarily interior Cold symptoms arise, such as aversion to cold and a feeling of cold, especially in the lower *jiao* (abdomen), the feet, knees and lower back due to the Kidney fire being too weak to warm the body.

Water: Kidney *yang* deficiency slows down the body metabolism, which leads to disorders within the fallopian tubes. This causes fluids to build up, leading to blockages of Phlegm and the growth of endometriosis.

As Kidney *yang* is involved in fluid metabolism, a deficiency will lead to fluid accumulation, causing puffiness and oedema, especially in the legs. There may be watery discharge, such as increased whitish vaginal discharge or watery ejaculate. The tongue can mirror this by becoming swollen and wet.

Urination: The amount and frequency of urination will vary according to, for example, the level of fluid intake, consumption of diuretic beverages (such as coffee) and the amount of perspiration. If Kidney *yang* is deficient the bladder is less able to metabolize fluids, which therefore accumulate, causing frequent clear urination. At night, when *yang* is at its weakest, nocturia (night-time urination) can be a problem.

Fertility: Disorders may arise with the movement and nourishment of the egg. The egg may be unable to travel through the fallopian tubes if the *yang* is too weak to provide movement. This weakness is also often at the root of ovulation disorders such as endometriosis or Polycystic Ovary Syndrome (PCOS). Kidney *yang* is also needed to maintain warmth within the womb during the post-ovulation phase (in Western terms the progesterone produced by the corpus luteum must be sufficient to keep the embryo in the uterus).

Sexual activity: Kidney essence and the warmth of Kidney *yang* nourish sexual energy. If Kidney *yang* is lacking, it will cause lack of libido, infertility in women and low BBT values in the luteal phase.

Bones: With Kidney *yang* deficiency, there is not enough *qi* to strengthen the bones and spinal column, resulting in backache and weakness of the legs and knees, which is aggravated by cold and rainy weather.

Sperm production: The sperm and its motility are associated with *yang*; Kidney *yang* deficiency leads to a reduction in the quality and quantity of sperm. In addition, *yang* is the source of warmth in the penis and the strength of erection and ejaculation; therefore if Kidney *yang* is weak it leads to impotence or the inability to sustain erection.

Treatment principle
Warming and supporting Kidney *yang*.

Typical acupuncture points and explanation
Guan Yuan (CV-4) and **Zhong Ji** (CV-3) may be used in combination with **Da He** (KID-12) to stimulate ovulation.

Ming Men (GV-4): can be used to regulate *yang qi*.

Qi Hai (CV-6) and **Guan Yuan** (CV-4): with moxa on the needle warm Kidney *yang*, tonify the Kidney and strengthen the uterus.

Tai Xi (KID-3): supplements Kidney *yang*.

Zhao Hai (KID-6): reinforces *yang* and has a warming function.

Leading herbal formula
You Gui Wan, Restore the right Kidney pill (see page 185).

Lifestyle and diet recommendations
Depending on the severity of the *yang* deficiency, warming foods and spices should be increased. The following tips will help to strengthen *yang*:

- Eat warm, cooked meals where possible.
- Use plenty of spices when cooking to promote the *yang* in your food.

- Choose plenty of easily digestible grains such as buckwheat or rice.
- Make sure meat and fish are lean.
- Include legumes, such as black beans, in your diet and lots of nuts and seeds.
- The cooking methods which are believed to increase *yang* are baking, roasting and slow braising.
- Avoid cold drinks or iced drinks taken straight out of the fridge.
- Too much banana, pear, cranberry or watermelon may increase the Cold in the body and slow down the metabolism and movement of fluids.
- See page 213 for a list of specific recommended foods.

Case study

Gillian, aged 35/Jon, aged 35

PROBLEMS:	**severe PCOS/severe male infertility**
METHODS TRIED:	**treatment for PCOS**
TCM OBJECTIVE:	**to improve Blood flow to the ovaries**
LENGTH OF TREATMENT:	**1½ years**
OUTCOME:	**natural conception; 3 children in the long term**

Jon and Gillian were in their mid-30s when they came to see us at The Zhai Clinic. Gillian had been diagnosed with Polycystic Ovary Syndrome (PCOS). Her menstrual cycle was severely prolonged, varying from 70 days to five months. She had been advised to take Metformin to reduce inflammation. After one year on Metformin, her cycle had reduced to 50 to 70 days. She was then advised to take Clomiphene (a drug that is used to induce ovulation) to help her to conceive. She had completed four cycles of Clomiphene ovulation induction by the time she approached us for TCM. Her cycle was between 30 and 45 days long during ovulation induction, but as yet, no pregnancy had been achieved. The couple was on the waiting list for free IVF treatment and they wanted to seek help from TCM to maximize their chances of success.

TCM assessment and treatment plan
The length of Gillian's menstrual cycle had been greatly reduced using the therapeutic Metformin management. However, the root of the problem of her prolonged menstrual cycle had not been well addressed. Her pulses were deep and difficult to feel altogether but there were no other obvious abnormalities.

I advised Gillian to continue with the Metformin management, but to stop the Clomiphene ovulation induction for the time being, until her ovarian performance had improved. In my experience, that would enable the TCM to work more effectively, by continuing to regulate her menstrual cycle, improve egg quality and encourage healthy fertilization. It would also allow the Clomiphene ovulation induction to work better when treatment was resumed.

TCM treatment in Gillian's case was designed to help improve Blood flow to her abdomen, which would benefit the ovary function, regulate the menstrual cycle and result in better egg quality. During her 13 months of TCM treatment, Gillian's menstrual cycle gradually reduced to 36 and then 35 days. As her cycle became more regular, I felt it would be a good time to begin helping her husband to improve his semen quality and quantity. He had a severely low sperm count.

During her husband's fourth month of TCM treatment, the couple's IVF appointment arrived. The fertility clinic they were attending was against Chinese medicine. The doctor told the couple to stop the Chinese medicine if they wanted to begin IVF. The couple told the consultant that they would not stop the TCM as they could see how much it had helped Gillian's menstrual cycles and she felt so much better and stronger in herself. The hospital delivered the results of Jon's latest semen analysis during the appointment, which showed the consultant clearly (much to his surprise) that both the quantity and quality of Jon's semen had much improved. The sperm count increased from 1 million to 19 million/ml; motility had increased from 60 per cent to 73 per cent; and forward progression had increased from 26 per cent to 35 per cent. He was speechless but still insisted that the couple should stop the TCM otherwise no treatment would be offered to them.

It was a big emotional struggle for the couple to decide whether or not to take the advice of the IVF clinic and potentially lose the IVF slot offered to them. The couple informed the clinic that they would not stop the TCM treatment during IVF and they would be responsible for themselves. The following month, with IVF about to start, Gillian discovered that she had conceived – there was no need for IVF!

We gave Gillian a herbal remedy to take immediately after the birth of her first child that would help her uterus to recover more effectively and to preserve her fertility levels. We were subsequently informed by the couple that they are now parents of three children. The second and the third pregnancies were spontaneous pregnancies achieved without any form of external help.

Chapter 8

A GUIDE TO CHINESE HERBS

There are thousands of standard formulas and variations in TCM that have been devised over hundreds of years and are used in very precise ways by qualified TCM practitioners. Plants are prepared, dried and processed in different ways, each of which has a different healing purpose. The herbal prescriptions included in this chapter stem from the TCM tradition, several of which I have modified successfully for the purpose of improving fertility in men and women.

Taking Chinese herbs

A TCM practitioner will give you your prescription in one of the following forms, all of which are equally effective, with directions for taking it. Your doctor will decide which method of preparation is best for your specific needs, whether it is in tablet, powder, liquid, granule or dry, loose form.

Boiled solution or decoction

A boiled solution or decoction is obtained by boiling the herbs with an appropriate amount of water for a fixed period of time. Boiling and decocting are the oldest forms of herbal prescription. The doctor selects the herbs he or she feels are appropriate for the patient, who will then take them home, soak them in water, boil them, strain them and drink as a 'tea'.

Many patients complain of how unpleasant and bitter herbal teas taste but most get used to it very quickly and even tell me that they come to like it.

Pills

The herbal mixture is pre-prepared by grinding the herbs into powder, mixing the powder with honey or other herbal juices and making round pills of various sizes.

Granules

Some practitioners prepare the herbal mixture by making an extract of the herbs, adding water and then rendering it into fine granules. The patient dissolves the granules in boiling water to take the medicine.

Powder

The herbs are ground into a fine powder, to be taken orally with water or rice soup. Some conditions may benefit from it being taken with rice wine.

Liquid

Liquid prescriptions have been pre-prepared by decocting one or more herbs in water, and reducing them (boiling them down) to a certain volume, or by making an extract of the herbs and dissolving it in water to form a solution.

Medical wine

The liquid is prepared by soaking the herbs in rice wine for a fixed period of time, then filtering out the residue. Traditionally, men drink it for maintaining general health and libido.

DRINKING HERBAL TEAS

If you find the tea difficult to drink, the best way is to wait until it has cooled down a bit. Then, while it is still warm, hold your nose and drink all the liquid at once, as quickly as possible. It is the smell of the tea that is the problem for some people: so as long as you don't smell it, it will be fine. I also find that rinsing the mouth with water afterwards may help, or perhaps eating a piece of dried fruit. But I *do not* recommend drinking water or juice immediately afterwards as this will dilute the effect of the herbal medicine.

THE INGREDIENTS

The beauty of Chinese herbals is that they can be used as a single ingredient or in composite form, in the following ways:

Minor prescriptions

These are low-dosage prescriptions containing a single herb or just a few different herbs that have a mild action. They are suitable for minor problems or sensitive individuals.

Mild prescriptions

These are composed of herbs that are moderate in action, used mainly in classical formulas (prescriptions), in pill form.

Composite prescriptions

These prescriptions are made by combining herbs in a unique formula, tailor-made for an individual. They generally combine several different remedies all in one prescription. My clinic uses composite prescriptions and we commission companies that specialize in manufacturing herbal pharmaceuticals to make them to our unique specification.

When we are designing a compound prescription, we must take into account the interactions between herbs. TCM doctors will compose a prescription that combines different herbs according to the needs of the person or disease and the therapeutic principle of TCM, while also bearing in mind the characteristics of the herbs themselves. Most Chinese herbal treatments use formulas containing approximately a dozen individual herbs which have been found to have a primary effect on one or more organ of the body.

Generally, there are four components to a compound prescription. These have been given various names, but the four functions remain the same:

1. **The principals** (monarch or chief) – these are the herbs that have the main therapeutic effect.

2. **The adjuvants** (minister or deputy) – these herbs assist or strengthen the effects of the principals.

3. **The assistants** (auxiliary or sometimes adjuvant) – these are herbs chosen to relieve secondary symptoms, to reduce complications or reduce the more extreme effects of the principal herbs.

4. **The messengers** (guide or conductor) – these are herbs that guide the actions of the herbs in the other three groups above to the affected region of the body. They also harmonize the effect of the prescription as a whole.

CAUTION

I always caution against self-diagnosis and treatment with Chinese herbal remedies because the sector is not regulated in the West. It is possible to buy anything over the internet these days and you will have absolutely no idea where the herbs originated or what else they may contain. Also, you may not be familiar with their effects. For example, Korean ginseng can boost energy and increase libido. However, it is not suitable for everyone as it may also cause side effects such as breathlessness, high blood pressure, Blood stagnation and Dampness. It is very important to ensure that you consult a properly qualified TCM practitioner before taking any kind of ginseng or other herbal medicine.

Case study

Marie-Therese, aged 37

PROBLEM:	**recurrent miscarriage, bleeding throughout pregnancy, severe psoriasis**
METHODS TRIED:	**natural conception**
TCM OBJECTIVE:	**to improve Blood circulation and clear psoriasis**
LENGTH OF TREATMENT:	**ongoing**
OUTCOME:	**3 children in the long term**

Marie-Therese was 37 years old when she came to see us. She had previously had three spontaneous pregnancies. The first miscarried at 12 weeks, the second unfortunately died inside the womb at 25 weeks and was surgically removed; her third pregnancy miscarried at 9 weeks. She had bled during all of her previous pregnancies.

Following the second unsuccessful pregnancy, she had developed severe psoriasis. Her whole body was covered with thick, itchy patches. Following surgery she experienced chills and fever. She suffered from constant lower abdominal pain and sweated a lot. Her periods were regular but extremely light. Her tongue was dull red, with many small, dull purple patches. Her pulse was choppy and deep.

TCM assessment and treatment plan

Marie-Therese's constitution was prone to Blood stasis. Her Blood circulation was poor and her body was unable to support the development of the pregnancy, even though she did not find it difficult to conceive. The surgical removal of her second pregnancy had traumatized her body, further injuring both vital energy and Blood. In TCM terms, there was an imbalance of *yin* and *yang*, which showed in the relationship between her Blood and *wei* (the disease on the skin at surface level). This resulted in psoriasis, the chills and fever after the surgery, and her frequent sweating. Marie-Therese understood that she needed help for her general health and had always consulted TCM practitioners, so it felt natural to turn to my clinic for help. By getting the Blood moving and improving her circulation we aimed to clear her psoriasis as much as possible and pave the way for a future healthly pregnancy. It was not a quick fix.

By the 16th month of TCM treatment, Marie-Therese's psoriasis condition had stabilized and was much less itchy; her abdominal pain was reduced, she no longer felt chills and fever and sweated less. Marie-Therese also discovered she was pregnant. Due to her previous bleeding during the pregnancy, we continued to support Marie-Therese with herbal medication into her ninth month of pregnancy. By then, her bleeding had completely stopped and she gave birth to a healthy girl at full term.

She chose to continue TCM treatment to give her support immediately after the birth. She went on to have two more pregnancies. Her second pregnancy used TCM support until the bleeding stopped at six months, and her third pregnancy used TCM support until the bleeding stopped at three months. All three pregnancies resulted in healthy babies.

Chinese herbal formulas (prescriptions)

The following are some examples of the herbal prescriptions that I use clinically with an explanation of how they work.

Xue Fu Zhu Yu Tang
Drive out stasis in the middle and lower abdomen tea

This prescription is used in the treatment of excessive Damp-Heat (see pages 147–151). It is designed to activate Blood circulation, remove Blood stasis and toxicity, promote the circulation of vital energy and relieve pain.

I have modified this classic TCM prescription to my own specification and use it mostly on patients who have been diagnosed with endometriosis, ovarian cysts, a history of ectopic pregnancy, partially blocked fallopian tubes and period pain due to Blood stasis.

MAIN INGREDIENTS

Tao Ren	Semen persicae	(Peach kernel)
Hong Hua	Flos carthami tinctorii	(Safflower)
Chi Shao Yao	Radix paeoniae rubra	(Red peony root)
Dang Gui	Radix angelicae sinensis	(Angelica root)
Gan Cao	Radix glychyrrhizae	(Liquorice root)
Sheng Di Huang	Radix rehmanniae glutinosae	(Chinese foxglove root)
Chuan Niu Xi	Radix cyathulae	(Cyanthula root)
Zhi Ke	Fructus citri seu ponciri	(Bitter orange root)
Chai Hu	Radix bupleuri	(Bupleurum root)

Tao Ren (Peach kernel) is used to activate Blood circulation and eliminate Blood stasis. It is very potent and is commonly used for gynaecological disorders such as menstrual pain, amenorrhea or irregular menstruation caused by Blood stasis.

Hong Hua (Safflower) and **Chi Shao Yao** (Red peony root) work with *Tao Ren* to activate Blood circulation and eliminate Blood stasis.

Dang Gui (Angelica root), also known as *Dong Quai*, is female ginseng. It nourishes and promotes Blood circulation and vital energy without injuring the *yin* Blood when dispelling Blood stasis.

Gan Cao (Liquorice root) reduces the more extreme effects of the principal herbs and harmonizes the action of all the herbs in this formula.

Sheng Di Huang (Chinese foxglove root) and **Chuan Niu Xi** (Cyanthula root) clear the Heat in the lower part of the body, encourage bowel movement and increase Blood flow downwards.

Zhi Ke (Bitter orange root) and **Chai Hu** (Bupleurum root) together smooth the flow of Liver *qi* to prevent future Liver *qi* stagnation.

Other possible additions

- **Bai Jiang Cao** (Patrinia) is a member of the Valerian family of herbs. It clears Heat and eliminates toxins and is used to eliminate Blood stasis and relieve pain. It is useful when treating those with a history of Pelvic Inflammatory Disease (PID).
- **Che Qian Zi** (Plantain seed) clears Heat and encourages urination to relieve urinary obstruction.

Xiao Yao Tang
Easy wanderer tea

I use this classic prescription to treat Liver *qi* stagnation (see pages 140–144). It has been designed to disperse the stagnation of Liver energy, strengthen the Spleen and nourish the Blood. We use this prescription widely in cases of stress-related problems such as painful distension of the stomach, dizziness, tiredness, poor appetite, sore breasts, premenstrual tension and bloated stomach.

MAIN INGREDIENTS

Chai Hu	*Radix bupleuri*	(Bupleurum root)
Dang Gui	*Radix angelicae sinensis*	(Angelica root)
Bai Zhu	*Rhizoma atractylodis macrocephalae*	(White atractylodes rhizome)

Bai Shao Yao	*Radix paeoniae lactiflorae*	(White peony root)
Fu Ling	*Sclerotium poriae cocos*	(Tuckahoe)
Zhi Gan Cao	*Radix glychyrrhizae uralensis*	(Honey-fried liquorice root)
Bo He	*Herba menthae*	(Mint)
Sheng Jiang	*Rhizoma zingiberis recens*	(Fresh ginger)

Chai Hu (Bupleurum root) is an important herb in the treatment of Liver *qi* stagnation as it moves *qi* and soothes the Liver.

Bai Shao Yao (White peony root) relaxes spasms and alleviates pain. Together with **Dang Gui** (Angelica root) it nourishes Liver Blood and soothes Liver function.

Bai Zhu (White atractylodes rhizome), together with **Fu Ling** (Tuckahoe), strengthens the Spleen and encourages the production of *qi* and Blood to increase vital energy.

Sheng Jiang (Fresh ginger) and **Bo He** (Mint) assist the other herbs in their action to strengthen the Spleen and sooth the Liver. **Zhi Gan Cao** (Honey-fried liquorice root) harmonizes the action of the other herbs in this formula. Used together, these herbs combine to ensure the normal functioning of the Liver and Spleen.

OTHER HERBS USED TO TREAT STAGNATED LIVER *QI*

Xiang Fu (Nut grass rhizome) is one of the most important herbs for the treatment of irregular menstruation and premenstrual syndrome arising from Liver *qi* stagnation.

Zhi Ke (Bitter orange root) mildly regulates *qi* and resolves stagnation to relieve congestion.

Xia Ku Cao (Prunella spike) is commonly used to clear Liver Fire. If there is Liver Fire with Blood deficiency, it is combined with **Dang Gui** (Angelica root), **Bai Shao Yao** (White peony root) and **Xuan Shen** (Figwort root), while for Liver *qi* stagnation it is used in combination with **Chai Hu** (Bupleurum root) and **Xiang Fu** (Nut grass rhizome).

Bai Shao Yao (White peony root) nourishes Blood and *yin*, softens the Liver and is an important herb to regulate menstruation and alleviate pain.

Bai Zhu (White atractylodes rhizome) tonifies Spleen *qi*, which nourishes the foetus and keeps it in the right place, thus calming the foetus and treating unstable pregnancy accompanied by Spleen *qi* deficiency.

Other possible additions

- **Mu Dan Pi** (Tree peony root) and **Shan Zhi Zi** (Gardenia fruit) reduce excessive Liver Heat.
- **Han Lian Cao** (False daisy) and **Nu Zhen Zi** (Privet fruit) nourish Liver and Kidney *yin*.
- **Wu Wei Zi** (Schisandra fruit) and **Sang Shen Zi** (Mulberry fruit) nourish the Liver Blood.
- **Shu Di Huang** (Steamed Chinese foxglove root) may be added to tonify Blood and nourish *yin*.
- **Sheng Di Huang** (Chinese foxglove root) may be added to clear Liver Heat and ease constipation.
- **He Huan Pi** (Mimosa tree bark) improves sleep pattern.

Liu Wei Di Huang Tang
Six flavour tea

This is a classic treatment for Kidney *yin* deficiency (see page 158–168). The formula consists of six herbs that combine to tonify Kidney *yin*, the vital energy for reproduction and providing the essential materials for egg and sperm production.

MAIN INGREDIENTS

Shu Di Huang	*Radix rehmanniae glutinosae conquitae*	(Steamed Chinese foxglove root)
Shan Yu Rou	*Fructus corni officinalis*	(Asiatic cornelian cherry fruit)
Huai Shan Yao	*Radix dioscorea oppositae*	(Chinese yam root)
Fu Ling	*Sclerotium poriae cocos*	(Tuckahoe)
Mu Dan Pi	*Cortex moutan radicis*	(Tree peony root)
Ze Xie	*Rhizoma alismatis*	(Water plantain root)

Shu Di Huang (Steamed Chinese foxglove root), **Shan Yu Rou** (Asiatic cornelian cherry fruit) and **Huai Shan Yao** (Chinese yam root) are potent herbs that reinforce *yin*.

Fu Ling (Tuckahoe), **Mu Dan Pi** (Tree peony root) and **Ze Xie** (Water plantain root) have a draining effect and prevent the rich, cloying properties of the principal herbs from causing congestion in the Kidneys and digestive system.

Other possible additions

This dependable formula, trusted by so many TCM practitioners, can be modified and used in many ways. For example:

- I often add **Zhi Mu** (Anemarrhena root) and **Huang Bai** (Cork tree bark) to enrich the *yin*, nourish the Kidneys and clear Damp-Heat. This is often known as *Zhi Bai Di Huang Tang* (Eight flavour tea), which is good for men with poor sperm production that presents as a combination of weak Kidney *yin* deficiency and Damp-Heat.
- Adding **Nu Zhen Zi** (Privet fruit) and **Han Lian Cao** (False daisy) to nourish Liver and Kidney *yin* and *jing*, will dispel deficient Heat. These two herbs also serve to nourish Kidney essence and help improve egg and sperm quality.
- By adding **Gou Qi Zi** (Wolf berry) and **Ju Hua** (Chrysanthemum flower), the mixture will clear Liver Heat and tonify Kidney *yin*. It effectively nourishes different parts of the body without creating stagnation and can be used for a prolonged period of time. This prescription is also famously used for poor vision or eyesight deficiency due to age; but equally, it helps the nourishment of Kidney *yin* and essence, which is good for the development of eggs and sperm.
- Adding **Wu Wei Zi** (Schisandra fruit) and **Tu Si Zi** (Chinese dodder) will warm Kidney *yang* and invigorate Kidney *yin*. This mixture is indicated for cases with a deficiency of both Kidney *yin* and Kidney *yang*. It is particularly useful to treat a man with a low sperm count and motility. It is also good for the development of eggs.

Tiao Jing Tang
Regulate the period tea

This formula is used to treat Blood and *qi* deficiency (see pages 155–158). It consists of several groups of herbs that nourish *qi* and Blood, soothe Liver *qi*, clear away Heat and move Blood stasis. It is used mainly for regulating the menstrual cycle in cases where there is an underlying health problem.

Tiao Jing Tang means to regulate the period. It refers to irregular periods that sometimes come early and sometimes late, and which may be accompanied by premenstrual tension, backache and/or scanty bleeding. This indicates Liver *qi* stagnation, Blood stasis, Kidney deficiency and/or Blood deficiency. In TCM terms, it is the Spleen that produces *qi* and Blood from ingested food and drink.

MAIN INGREDIENTS

Shu Di Huang	*Radix rehmanniae glutinosae conquitae*	(Steamed Chinese foxglove root)
Huang Qi	*Radix astragali*	(Astragalus)

Dang Shen	*Radix codonopsis pilosulae*	(Codonopsis root)
Bai Shao Yao	*Radix paeoniae lactiflorae*	(White peony root)
Dang Gui	*Radix angelicae sinensis*	(Angelica root)
Dan Shen	*Radix salviae miltiorrhizae*	(Salvia root)
Xiang Fu	*Rhizoma cyperi rotundi*	(Nut grass rhizome)
Bai Zhu	*Rhizoma atractylodis macrocephalae*	(White atractylodes rhizome)
Tian Dong	*Tuber asparagi*	(Asparagus root)
Huai Shan Yao	*Radix dioscorea oppositae*	(Chinese yam root)

Huang Qi (Astragalus), **Dang Shen** (Codonopsis root), **Bai Zhu** (White atractylodes rhizome) and **Huai Shan Yao** (Chinese yam root) combine to nourish the *qi*. Together they strengthen the Spleen and are therefore essential herbs to support the Spleen in its function to supply *qi* and Blood.

Shu Di Huang (Steamed Chinese foxglove root) and **Bai Shao Yao** (White peony root) invigorate the Blood. *Shu Di Huang* strengthens the Liver and Kidneys and generates essence (*jing*). It is a very good herb for tonifying the Blood and it is said to nourish the *yin* of the Blood. This herb is particularly effective in treating problems with menstruation, conception and birth. **Dang Gui** (Angelica root) invigorates the Blood and is said to nourish *yang*.

Tian Dong (Asparagus root) nourishes the Blood and nourishes the Lung to improve Kidney *yin* and clear any Heat generated as a result of *yin* deficiency. **Dan Shen** (Salvia root) invigorates the Blood, dispels stasis and promotes the production of new Blood, while **Xiang Fu** (Nut grass rhizome) harmonizes the Liver *qi*. It is an essential herb in treating irregular menstruation and pain due to Blood stasis.

Bu Yin Jian
Tea to reinforce yin

Bu Yin decoction was created by Zhang Jingyue (1583–1640) a famous physician who was practising TCM during the Ming Dynasty. It is used to treat Kidney *yin* deficiency Heat (see pages 158–162), when complicated by some *yang* deficiency, Liver depression and possibly some Blood stasis. It is composed of eight herbs which tonify and cool Blood, nourish *yin* and calm the foetus.

The formula is often used in cases where there is the threat of miscarriage; where there is vaginal bleeding, a dry mouth, a red tongue with a thin and yellow coating, and a small and rapid pulse. At my clinic, we may use this prescription to prevent miscarriage and to support the pregnancy until a woman has reached the three-month point.

MAIN INGREDIENTS

Sheng Di Huang	*Radix rehmanniae glutinosae*	(Chinese foxglove root)
Shu Di Huang	*Radix rehmanniae glutinosae conquitae*	(Steamed Chinese foxglove root)
Bai Shao Yao	*Radix paeoniae lactiflorae*	(White peony root)
Huai Shan Yao	*Radix dioscorea oppositae*	(Chinese yam root)
Huang Qin	*Radix scutellariae baicalensis*	(Scutellaria)
Huang Bai	*Cortex phellodendri*	(Cork tree bark)
Xu Duan	*Radix dipsaci*	(Japanese teasel root)
Gan Cao	*Radix glychyrrhizae*	(Liquorice root)

Shu Di Huang (Steamed Chinese foxglove root) strongly nourishes essence and Kidney *yin*, while **Sheng Di Huang** (Chinese foxglove root) nourishes *yin*, clears Heat and cools the Blood.

Bai Shao Yao (White peony root) nourishes Liver Blood and **Huai Shan Yao** (Chinese yam root) supplements the *qi* of the Spleen and Kidney.

Huang Bai (Cork tree bark) and **Huang Qin** (Scutellaria) clear Heat, particularly in the lower and upper *jiao* (abdomen). **Xu Duan** (Japanese teasel root) warms *yang*, promotes Blood circulation and benefits the uterus. **Gan Cao** (Liquorice root) harmonizes the action of the other herbs in this formula.

Other possible additions

- The addition of **Chai Hu** (Bupleurum root) and **Zhi Shi** (Unripe bitter orange) will motivate the Liver *qi* to support the Kidney function.
- **Tu Si Zi** (Chinese dodder) and **Gou Qi Zi** (Wolf berry) nourish Kidney *yin* and essence and promote ovulation.
- The addition of **Nu Zhen Zi** (Privet fruit) and **Han Lian Cao** (False daisy) will help to nourish Kidney *yin*.
- **Bai Mao Gen** (Imperata) cools the Blood, stops bleeding and calms the foetus, which is particularly important during the early pregnancy.

- I add **Du Zhong** (Eucommia Bark) when there is a need to tonify Kidney *yang*, nourish the Liver and invigorate the Kidneys.
- **Wu Wei Zi** (Schisandra fruit) restrains essence and prevents excessive sweating.

Bi Xie Fen Qing Tang
Draining Dampness tea

My modification of this classic formula is designed to clear away Damp-Heat (see pages 147–151) in the lower part of body, by activating Blood circulation and eliminating toxic material. It is very useful for clearing a thick, yellow coating on the tongue and a wiry and rapid pulse. I find it very effective for treating male infertility.

Damp attributed to toxic material moving downwards to the lower abdomen may stay there for a long period of time, particularly around the testicles in men. This may be associated with Heat, caused by excessive alcohol intake and poor diet. This will create obstruction and blocks the movement of *qi*, sometimes causing an accumulation of Blood stasis, depending on the nature or constitution of the person.

The condition causes heaviness due to Damp and toxic Heat, which often suppresses the environment of the lower abdomen, making it difficult for the organs to function normally. Consequently, there is an impact on sperm production in men, and other associated problems.

MAIN INGREDIENTS

Bi Xie	*Rhizoma dioscorea*	(Yam rhizome)
Shi Chang Pu	*Rhizoma acori graminei*	(Sweet flag rhizome)
Huang Bai	*Cortex phellodendri*	(Cork tree bark)
Fu Ling	*Sclerotium poriae cocos*	(Tuckahoe)
Bai Zhu	*Rhizoma atractylodis macrocephalae*	(White atractylodes rhizome)
Lian Zi Xin	*Plumula nelumbinis nuciferae*	(Lotus plumule)
Mu Dan Pi	*Cortex moutan radicis*	(Tree peony root)
Ze Xie	*Rhizoma alismatis*	(Water plantain root)

Bi Xie (Yam rhizome) clears away Dampness and relaxes the tendons. It is the main herb used for clearing excessive Damp and Heat. It is very effective in the treatment of male infertility as the Damp often stays in the lower part of the body around the testicles.

Huang Bai (Cork tree bark) clears away Dampness and Heat and purges the Fire, while **Ze Xie** (Water plantain root) and **Fu Ling** (Tuckahoe) promote energy and clear away the Heat and Dampness. **Mu Dan Pi** (Tree peony root) cools the Blood and removes toxins when it combines with *Huang Bai* (Cork tree bark). It can also dredge the vessels and meridians when it combines with *Bi Xie* (Yam rhizome).

Tao Hong Si Wu Tang
Four herb decoction with safflower and peach kernel

This prescription is used to clear Blood stasis (see pages 137–140).

MAIN INGREDIENTS

Tao Ren	*Semen persicae*	(Peach kernel)
Hong Hua	*Flos carthami tinctorii*	(Safflower)
Dang Gui	*Radix angelicae sinensis*	(Angelica root)
Chi Shao Yao	*Radix paeoniae rubra*	(Red peony root)
Chuan Xiong	*Radix ligustici chuanxiong*	(Szechuan lovage root)
Shu Di Huang	*Radix rehmanniae glutinosae conquitae*	(Steamed Chinese foxglove root)

Tao Ren (Peach kernel) and **Hong Hua** (Safflower) are potent herbs used to activate Blood circulation and eliminate Blood stasis. **Chuan Xiong** (Szechuan lovage root) tonifies the Blood, promoting improved circulation and vital energy. **Shu Di Huang** (Steamed Chinese foxglove root) and **Dang Gui** (Angelica root) nourish the Blood, and increase the Blood volume to dispel Blood stasis without injuring the *yin* and Blood.

Other possible additions

- **Chuan Niu Xi** (Cyanthula root) dispels Damp-Heat and Blood stagnation.
- **Zhi Ke** (Bitter orange root) promotes the movement of *qi*, to facilitate the movement of Blood.
- **Ai Ye** (Mugwort leaf) warms the uterus when there is Cold and improves Blood circulation.
- **Tu Si Zi** (Chinese dodder), **Gou Qi Zi** (Wolf berry), **Wu Wei Zi** (Schisandra fruit), **Fu Pen Zi** (Chinese raspberry) and **Che Qian Zi** (plantain seed) promote Kidney essence to provide fertility.

Qi Gong San
Arousing the uterus

This prescription is used to treat excessive Phlegm-Damp (see pages 144–147).
Its main function is to eliminate Dampness and, secondarily, to move *qi*, Blood and
stagnant food.

MAIN INGREDIENTS

Ban Xia	*Rhizoma pinelliae ternatae*	(Pinellia root)
Chen Pi	*Pericarpium citri reticulatae*	(Tangerine peel)
Cang Zhu	Rhizoma atractylodis *lanceae*	(Atractylodes)
Shen Qu	*Massa fermentata medicinalis*	(Medicated leaven)
Xiang Fu	*Rhizoma cyperi rotundi*	(Nut grass rhizome)
Chuan Xiong	*Radix ligustici chuanxiong*	(Szechuan lovage root)
Fu Ling	*Sclerotium poriae cocos*	(Tuckahoe)

Ban Xia (Pinellia root), **Chen Pi** (Tangerine peel), **Cang Zhu** (Atractylodes) and **Fu
Ling** (Tuckahoe) eliminate Dampness. **Shen Qu** (Medicated leaven) resolves food
accumulation, which eliminates Dampness. **Xiang Fu** (Nut grass rhizome) and **Chuan
Xiong** (Szechuan lovage root) move *qi* and Blood respectively, which also helps to
resolve Dampness.

Other possible additions

- **Hou Po** (Magnolia bark) lifts the *yang* with its special aroma. It moves *qi* and
  transforms Dampness.
- **Xu Duan** (Japanese teasel root) and **Tu Si Zi** (Chinese dodder) nourish and
  strength the Kidneys.
- **Dang Shen** (Codonopsis root) and **Shi Chang Pu** (Sweet flag rhizome) may be
  added if the patient is feeling tired.
- **Chuan Xiong** (Szechuan lovage root) and **Dang Gui** (Angelica root) activate
  Blood circulation when Phlegm has caused Blood stasis.

Gui Zhi Fu Ling Tang
Cinnamon twig and poria decoction

This is a classic prescription used primarily for treating an accumulation of Blood stasis in the womb, repeated miscarriage, infertility, postpartum bleeding, ovarian cysts, dysmenorrhea, endometriosis, irregular menstruation and fallopian tube blockage by Cold and Damp.

MAIN INGREDIENTS

Gui Zhi	*Ramulus cinnamomi cassiae*	(Cinnamon bark)
Fu Ling	*Sclerotium poriae cocos*	(Tuckahoe)
Bai Shao Yao	*Radix dioscorea oppositae*	(White peony root)
Mu Dan Pi	*Cortex moutan radicis*	(Tree peony root)
Tao Ren	*Semen persicae*	(Peach kernel)

This formula promotes Blood circulation, and helps to remove Blood stasis and blockages. **Gui Zhi** (Cinnamon bark) warms the Blood and unblocks Blood vessels, thereby reducing Blood stasis by promoting circulation. **Fu Ling** (Tuckahoe) transforms Phlegm and Dampness, which can complicate Blood stasis. In addition, *Fu Ling* (Tuckahoe) calms the mind to sooth pain. **Bai Shao Yao** (White peony root) protects *yin*, regulates Blood flow and relieves spasm and pain. **Mu Dan Pi** (Tree peony root) and **Tao Ren** (Peach kernel) transform Blood stasis and clear any Heat that may have developed.

Other possible additions

The herbs listed below may be added to the prescription to tonify *yang*, warm the womb and expel Cold:

- **Ba Ji Tian** (Morinda root) warms and fortifies Kidney *yang* and expels Cold Dampness.
- **Yin Yang Huo** (Epimedium) warms and fortifies Kidney *yang*, expels Cold Dampness and regulates *yin* and *yang*.
- **Ai Ye** (Mugwort leaf) warms the womb, disperses Cold and alleviates pain.
- **Rou Gui** (Chinese cassia bark) warms the Kidneys and meridians, tonifies *yang* and disperses Cold.

Qing Jing Tang
Clear the menses formula

This is a time-tested prescription commonly used for menstrual disorders caused by excessive Blood Heat.

MAIN INGREDIENTS

Sheng Di Huang	*Radix rehmanniae glutinosae*	(Chinese foxglove root)
Bai Shao Yao	*Radix paeoniae lactiflorae*	(White peony root)
Xuan Shen	*Radix scrophulariae ningpoensis*	(Figwort root)
Mai Men Dong	*Tuber ophiopogonis japonici*	(Ophiopogon root)
Jin Yin Hua	*Flos lonicerae japonicae*	(Honeysuckle flower)
Lian Qiao	*Fructus forsythiae suspensae*	(Forsythia fruit)
Huang Lian	*Rhizome coptidis*	(Goldthread root)
Dan Zhu Ye	*Herba lophatheri gracilis*	(Bamboo leaf)

Sheng Di Huang (Chinese foxglove root) and **Mai Men Dong** (Ophiopogon root) nourish *yin* and cool the Blood. **Bai Shao Yao** calms the Blood to help stop excessive bleeding. **Jin Yin Hua** (Honeysuckle flower), **Lian Qiao** (Forsythia fruit), **Huang Lian** (Goldthread root), **Xuan Shen** (Figwort root) and **Dan Zhu Ye** (Bamboo leaf) clear toxic Fire and dissipate nodules and Damp, to cool Blood and regulate menstruation.

You Gui Wan
Restore the right Kidney pill

This prescription is used to treat Kidney *yang* deficiency (see page 164–167). It is designed to tonify Kidney *yang*, but also nourishes Blood and benefits the Conception Vessel (*Ren mai*) (see page 51). It is called the 'right Kidney' pill because in TCM it is believed that *yang* warmth comes from the right Kidney. (*Yin* is associated with the left Kidney.)

MAIN INGREDIENTS

Shu Di Huang	*Radix rehmanniae glutinosae conquitae*	(Steamed Chinese foxglove root)
Tu Si Zi	*Semen cuscutae*	(Chinese dodder)
Huai Shao Yao	*Radix dioscorea oppositae*	(Chinese yam root)
Gou Qi Zi	*Fructus lycii chinensis*	(Wolf berry)
Dang Gui	*Radix angelicae sinensis*	(Angelica root)
Shan Yu Rou	*Fructus corni officinalis*	(Asiatic cornelian cherry fruit)
Du Zhong	*Cortex eucommiae ulmoidis*	(Eucommia bark)
Rou Gui	*Cortex cinnamomi cassiae*	(Chinese cassia bark)

Du Zhong (Eucommia bark) and **Tu Si Zi** (Chinese dodder) tonify and warm Kidney *yang*, while **Rou Gui** (Chinese cassia bark) warms the Kidneys and expels cold. **Shu Di Huang** (Steamed Chinese foxglove root), **Huai Shao Yao** (Chinese yam root) and **Shan Yu Rou** (Asiatic cornelian cherry fruit) supplement and firm the Kidneys, while **Dang Gui** (Angelica root) and **Gou Qi Zi** (Wolf berry) nourish the Blood and the Liver.

Other possible additions

- **Xiang Fu** (Nut grass rhizome) and **Zhi Ke** (Bitter orange root) are added to the prescription if there is abdominal distension.

Herbs to support and maintain a healthy pregnancy

Some herbs are particularly useful during early pregnancy and are important when there has been a history of miscarriage.

Ai Ye

Folium artemisiae argyi

(Mugwort leaf)

Ai Ye warms the womb and prevents bleeding. It calms the growing baby and may be recommended to patients under threat of miscarriage. It is used together with other ingredients such as *Chuan Xiong* (Szechuan lovage root) to repair the Conception and Penetrating Vessels (see pages 51–52), which run centrally down the front and back of the body. These two meridians closely influence pregnancy.

Bai Zhu

Rhizoma atractylodis macrocephalae

(White atractylodes rhizome)

This is used to treat the threat of miscarriage due to deficient Spleen *qi*, which is unable to support the Blood or nourish the foetus during the pregnancy.

Bai Mao Gen

Rhizoma Imperatae Cylindricae

(Imperata)

Bai Mao Gen cools the Blood. It is prescribed when there is bleeding caused by Heat in the Blood, especially in the lower *jiao* (abdomen), leading to pregnancy disorders.

Ban Xia

Rhizoma pinelliae ternatae

(Pinellia root)

This plant is slightly toxic so should usually be avoided during pregnancy. However, it can be detoxified for clinical use. The detoxified version is known as **Fa Ban Xia** (Prepared Pinellia root) and is very effective at harmonizing the stomach to relieve nausea and vomiting, and calming the digestive system. Therefore, women who suffer from nausea and vomiting during pregnancy are prescribed Fa Ban Xia.

Chuan Xiong

Radix ligustici chuanxiong

(Szechuan lovage root)

Chuan Xiong is slightly toxic so should be used with caution and avoided once pregnant. It promotes the flow of Blood and *qi* and relieves pain. It is used to treat gynaecological disorders such as irregular periods, amenorrhea, painful periods, difficult labour, postpartum abdominal pain, postpartum discharge or pain and swelling due to traumatic injury.

Huang Qin

Radix scutellariae baicalensis
(Scutellaria)
Huang Qin calms the foetus and is used where there is a risk of miscarriage due to toxic Heat.

Sha Ren

Amomum xanthoides
(Cardamom seed)
Sha Ren strengthens and warms the Spleen to promote the movement of *qi* and the transformation of Dampness to relieve morning sickness. Sha Ren also stabilizes pregnancy by calming the foetus.

Xu Duan

Radix dipsaci
(Japanese teasel root)
This reinforces the Liver and Kidneys, calms the foetus and stops uterine bleeding. Xu Duan is prescribed where there is a risk of miscarriage due to Kidney deficiency or bleeding during pregnancy. It is also used to treat heavy periods and bleeding between periods.

HERBS TO BE AVOIDED DURING PREGNANCY
IMPORTANT

When you become pregnant, it is very important to inform your TCM doctor immediately as certain herbs may need to be stopped or new herbs introduced to enable others to take effect. Some Chinese herbs, like conventional Western medicines, have contraindications, meaning that in some circumstances they should not be taken because there is a risk of adverse effects.

The very herbs that have a deep cleansing impact on the womb and can encourage implantation to take place may also work against the foetus once a woman becomes pregnant. Examples include herbs that activate Blood circulation and eliminate Blood stasis, including:

Tao Ren (Peach kernel)

Hong Hua (Safflower)

Chuan Xiong (Szechuan lovage root)

Chi Shao Yao (Red peony root)

In my experience I have found these herbs to be very good at improving endometrial health, as they promote healthy blood flow and dispel blood clots. These are the very herbs that encourage implantation to take place. I use them up to the fifth week of pregnancy in most cases, then change to other herbs from that point on.

However, they need to be used very carefully. If not used appropriately, they could harm the mother or developing baby during a pregnancy, or even induce miscarriage. That is another reason why it is very important to only ever take advice from a professionally qualified TCM doctor.

PART 4

Self-Help with Traditional Chinese Medicine

Chapter 9
EATING FOR FERTILITY

Eating a healthy diet is essential for both women and men – especially when you are trying to conceive. It is not only the woman who needs to keep her body in peak condition to conceive and nourish a developing baby; the man, too, needs to stay nutrition-conscious, in order to keep sperm production at optimum levels.

The human body needs the right fuels. It is crucial to eat foods that contain the right nutritional balance of vitamins, minerals, essential fatty acids, proteins and carbohydrates so the body can grow and function effectively. When you become pregnant, you carry and sustain new life inside your body. It is therefore vital to eat well and carefully, to ensure all the organs of your body are maintained in peak condition. This does not mean becoming obsessive or faddy about what you eat, you simply need to adopt common sense and an understanding of the basics of nutritional health.

Eating healthily is all about moderation and common sense. A healthy diet consists of a eating a balance of fresh vegetables and fruit, slow-release carbohydrates such as whole grains and pulses, and proteins such as chicken or fish, at every meal – together with lots of fibre and water. Eaten together, they are digested more slowly, and release a steady flow of energy that keeps the body feeling satisfied for longer. This is never more important than when you are trying to get pregnant.

Refined foods generally contain fewer natural nutrients. They are often supplemented with extra vitamins and minerals simply because the process of refining them has taken most of the goodness out.

Look after your digestive health
We all know that eating the right foods is important for general wellbeing; but not everyone realizes how important it is to look after the digestive system in particular. The digestive system is the gateway to health. It needs to be maintained in an excellent condition because it metabolizes and delivers nutrients to every organ of the body.

Keeping the digestive fluids in a healthy state ensures that the foods we eat can be easily broken down and the body can absorb the nutrients needed to maintain good health. We therefore need to avoid foods and drinks that could inflame or irritate the digestive system, such as iced or chilled drinks straight from the fridge, or foods that are very stimulating, such as alcohol, chilli or curry, because they can cause extreme damage to digestive fluids.

DON'T BE TOO STRICT

Food is a pleasure to be enjoyed. As long as the majority of our meals (say 80 per cent) consist of commonly recognized healthy foods, the occasional indulgent treat won't do much harm – even if you are pregnant.

Healthy eating for pregnancy

I normally advise patients to buy fresh food, particularly fruits and vegetables. The fresher the food, the greater the concentration of nutrients it will retain. When foods are stored for too long, some nutrients begin to oxidize and lose their nutritional value. It is usually preferable to buy organic products where possible and to buy them only in small quantities rather than stocking up too far in advance. However, above all, choose the freshest produce, even when there is a choice between organic and non-organic.

When a woman is trying to become pregnant, her diet should include the following:

PROTEIN

Every tissue in the body contains a high level of protein of some kind. Protein forms skin and muscle, helps in the production of amino acids and repairs cells. We need approximately 70–100 grams per day. A woman who is pregnant or trying to become pregnant may need more (about 140–200 grams) as there are extra heavy demands put on her body to provide for the development of the uterus and placenta (and in due course, the developing baby). Women who exercise a great deal or who undertake heavy physical work will definitely need to increase their protein intake.

Sources
- Poultry, meat and fish are important sources of protein. Game (such as partridge, venison and rabbit) will contain an even higher percentage of protein because it contains less fat.
- Dairy products, eggs.
- Pulses such as black-eyed beans, chickpeas, broad beans, baked beans and red, white or black beans.
- Nuts. These should be eaten in small amounts as they also contain a lot of fat.

CALCIUM

Calcium is necessary for the healthy formation of bones, nails and teeth and the correct functioning of nerves and muscles, including the heart muscle. Calcium also helps to prevent blood clots and provides vital nutrients for the development of a growing baby.

Sources

Calcium is present in a very wide range of foods. Overall, shellfish, grains and dairy products have the highest levels of calcium.

- Dairy products such as yogurt, milk and cheese.
- Calcium-fortified foods such as soy milk, bread and cereals.
- Dark green leafy vegetables.
- Eggs, seeds, nuts and pulses.
- Meat and fish, but only in moderate amounts (apart from chicken or fish stock, which has usually been made from calcium-rich bones). Canned fish that includes soft bones (such as sardines and salmon) are also a good source.

IRON

Iron helps defend the body against infections or inflammation and is needed for the metabolism of B vitamins. It helps to increase blood volume and prevent anaemia. Women are more prone to anaemia than men because of the monthly loss of blood associated with menstrual periods or fibroids. Iron is also an essential component of haemoglobin in the blood (in combination with sodium, potassium and water), which transports oxygen from the lungs to the organs of the body.

Sources

- Beef, pork, liver and poultry. The iron found in meat is most easily absorbed by the human body.
- Vegetables, particularly dark green leafy vegetables such as spinach.
- Whole grains, such as wholegrain bread and pasta, brown rice, porridge and breakfast cereals.
- Fish and seafood.
- Dried beans and pulses.
- Dried fruits, including dried apricots and raisins, and nuts.

VITAMIN C

Vitamin C is known to enhance immunity from infection and is an important element in the production of haemoglobin. It also acts as a detoxifier and protects tissues from damage. It helps to build a healthy immune system and is a vital component of body and bone development.

However, vitamin C is a fragile substance that is easily destroyed by heat during cooking and prolonged storage. Therefore, I would recommend buying fruits and vegetables in small quantities and eating them as fresh as possible.

Sources

- Fresh green vegetables, particularly leafy greens, broccoli and Brussels sprouts.
- Sweet peppers and sweet potatoes are also good sources.
- Most fruits are rich in vitamin C, particularly kiwi fruits and citrus fruits, such as lemons, limes and oranges.

START THE DAY WITH A CITRUS BOOST

Try starting each morning by drinking a cup of warm or hot water with a slice of fresh lemon and a little honey. The lemon will help to refresh your digestive system and give you a boost of vitamin C at the same time.

FOLIC ACID/FOLATES

Folic acid is a B vitamin which is often lacking in the diet. Folates (the natural form of folic acid) are needed for cell growth and blood production. The growing foetus will draw folates from the mother's blood so supplementation is usually important when you are trying to get pregnant, and during the pregnancy.

Folic acid plays a key role in reducing the risk of neural tube defects – serious birth defects of the brain and spine, such as spina bifida. All women trying for a baby should take a daily supplement of folic acid, from the time you stop using contraception until at least the 12th week of pregnancy, to help prevent birth defects. See pages 196–197 for advice about supplements.

Sources

- Green leafy vegetables, beans, peas, raw spinach and asparagus.
- Whole grains, such as brown rice, enriched breads, pasta and lentils.
- Fruits such as oranges, grapefruit and pineapple.
- Fortified bread and breakfast cereals.

FATS

Fat is essential in the diet because it transports the fat-soluble vitamins A, D, E and K around the body. There are two main types of fat found in food: unsaturated fats (these are the 'good' fats) and saturated fats (these are the 'bad' fats). They both contain the same amount of calories but we should cut down on foods that are high in saturated fat because they contribute towards a greater risk of developing cardiovascular disease and other health problems.

Good fats

Unsaturated fats can be divided into monounsaturated and polyunsaturated fats, which include omega-3 fatty acids. Unsaturated fats are liquid at room temperature and play an important role in keeping us healthy and reducing cholesterol levels. They are a vital source of essential fatty acids (EFAs) used in the formation of hormones, brain and nerve tissue. Good fats are rich in fat-soluble vitamins, such as vitamin A, D, E, K and pro-vitamins (which can be converted into vitamins in the body.)

Monounsaturated fats are found in high concentrations in peanuts, almonds, hazelnuts and pecans, olives and avocados. Other sources include olive oil and seeds such as pumpkin and sesame.

Polyunsaturated fats are found mostly in green leafy vegetables, nuts, seeds and fish. Natural, unprocessed foods are always the healthiest choice.

OMEGA-3 FATS

Omega-3 fats are polyunsaturated fats and are essential for maintaining the healthy production of hormones and helping to regulate many important physiological functions including blood clotting, blood pressure and the healthy functioning of the nervous system.

Omega-3 fats are found in oily fish. The best sources are cold-water fish such as tuna, sardines, anchovies, herring and salmon. There are also vegetable sources (for example, flax oil), but they are much less efficient and need to be eaten in far larger quantities.

The body requires more omega-3 fatty acids when it is under stress, suffering from disease or when the weather is cold or the climate lacks sunshine. A good-quality supplement from a reputable manufacturer can be very effective and can be beneficial for those on a vegetarian diet.

Sources
- Oily fish such as salmon, mackerel, herring, pilchards, sardines, trout and fresh tuna.
- Flax oil or omega-3 enriched oils.
- Avocados, nuts and seeds (almonds, cashews, hazelnuts, walnuts, pine nuts, sesame seeds, sunflower seeds, peanuts and pistachios).
- Olive oil and other oils including rapeseed oil, corn oil and sunflower oil.
- Lean meats.
- Green leafy vegetables.
- Skimmed or semi-skimmed milk and low-fat cheeses.

Bad fats
Saturated fats are the 'bad' fats and should be eaten only in small quantities. They are found in butter, hard cheeses, whole milk, fatty meats and meat products such as sausages, cream, ice cream, mayonnaise, lard, dripping, suet, ghee, coconut oil and palm oil. Saturated fats are generally solid at room temperature.

Choose lean, unprocessed meats and opt for grilling, baking or steaming, whatever you are cooking, rather than frying or roasting.

BEWARE OF TRANS-FATS

One group of fats should be avoided completely if possible. These are called trans-fats. There are both trans-unsaturated and trans-saturated foods on the market. They are artificial, hydrogenated fats that are often used in processed foods to prolong their shelf life – this includes 'comfort' foods such as biscuits, pies, cakes, chocolate, crackers, fried foods, takeaways and pastries. Trans-fats have little or no nutritional benefit. If you can't avoid them completely, eat them only in very small amounts and very occasionally.

WATER

Water is an essential nutrient. There is much talk about the importance of drinking 2 or 3 litres of water a day, but I believe it is unwise to generalize. Everyone has different needs, which depend on their personal constitution, lifestyle and their body's requirements. One useful way to monitor and adjust whether you are drinking enough water is by checking the colour and concentration of your urine. If your urine is very yellow or dark you need to drink more water as urine should be pale, clear and odourless.

During a TCM consultation, we often ask our patients whether or not they feel thirsty. Some patients feel thirsty but do not feel like a drink (this indicates *yin* deficiency but without too much body Heat); others feel thirsty and drink a lot and also like cold drinks (which suggests Heat or Fire in the body). Everyone's diagnosis is different. However, it is true that most of us don't drink enough during a normal day, so a good rule of thumb is to drink slightly more than you think you need.

Take care Excessive water intake can cause sodium levels in the blood stream to fall, and in extreme cases even lead to death. The 'right' level of water intake varies from person to person, which is why I tend not to specify a particular quantity. In general I recommend that people drink the amount of water that they feel like consuming – or just slightly more. For example, if you tend to feel like drinking four glasses of water a day, perhaps drink five glasses – but not more than that.

Sources

Water is present in all foods, especially fruit and vegetables. However, a glass of fresh water is the best source. Whether you prefer tap water, bottled water, still, sparkling, warm or cool is up to you. However, it is best to avoid very hot or very cold water, as this will shock your stomach and your digestive system.

Vitamin and mineral supplements

Vitamins and minerals are a vital part of your daily diet, essential for body and organ health. If your daily diet is well balanced and consists of a variety of fresh fruits, vegetables, whole grains, chicken, fish, eggs and seeds, you will probably be receiving sufficient vitamins and minerals. It is unlikely that you could ever consume more nutrients than your body can handle through eating natural foods, except by eating a large quantity of iron-rich offal, such as liver.

However, many of the foods we eat are heavily processed or have been stored for a long time, which means their mineral and vitamin content will have been reduced. This is why I recommend introducing just a small quantity of essential supplements to support the body in case the food we eat has lost its nutrients during cooking or storage.

TAKE CARE

Vitamin and mineral supplements should always be treated with caution and respect. Always read the labels and never exceed the recommended dosage. This is because supplements contain high doses in concentrated form, which could be dangerous or may overload the body's organs if taken in excessive or inappropriate amounts.

Measurements and abbreviations:

μg or mcg = micrograms

mg = milligrams

g = grams

There are 1,000 micrograms in 1 milligram

There are 1,000 milligrams in 1 gram

SUPPLEMENTS FOR WOMEN

Folic acid

The recommended daily allowance (RDA) of folic acid is between 400 and 800 mcg (micrograms). If you decide to take your folic acid in a multi-vitamin supplement, make sure it contains 400 mcg folic acid and does not contain vitamin A as too much could harm your baby and cause birth defects.

If you have been pregnant before and suffered a neural tube defect or if you have diabetes, it is advisable to ask your healthcare professional for further advice. Doctors may send you for further tests or recommend that you take an increased level of folic acid: up to 5,000 mcg per day. You will need a prescription for this higher dose.

You may be prescribed a larger dose if:

- You have previously had a baby with spina bifida
- You have coeliac disease
- You have diabetes
- You are taking medicine for epilepsy

It is important to take medical advice, rather than to self-diagnose.

Vitamin D

Vitamin D works with calcium and is essential for the creation of strong, healthy bones and protection against DNA damage.

The RDA for vitamin D is 5 mcg. The best source is sunlight, because the body naturally converts sunlight into vitamin D. Very few foods contain vitamin D, apart from oily fish, fortified margarines and some breakfast cereals, but supplements are available.

Vitamin C

Vitamin C (also known as ascorbic acid) is one of the antioxidant vitamins. It is vital for iron absorption, amino acid metabolism, healthy skin and eyes and boosting the immune system. The RDA for vitamin C is 40–80 mg. It cannot be stored in the body, so it needs to be replenished daily. See page 193 for a list of dietary sources.

Iron

Iron is carried in the red blood cells where it helps carry oxygen and is also essential to keep the immune system healthy. Low iron levels have been linked to tiredness and can contribute to a failure to ovulate. Women need about 15 mg of iron per day. Vitamin C is needed to help absorb iron so try to combine them in a meal or supplement. See page 192 for a list of dietary sources.

Calcium

Calcium is the most important mineral for building healthy bones and teeth in the mother and the developing foetus. It also helps blood to clot and muscles to contract. It regulates nerve function and blood pressure and the secretion of hormones. We need about 700 mg of calcium per day. Vitamin D is needed to help absorb calcium so try to combine them in a meal or supplement. See page 192 for a list of dietary sources.

SUPPLEMENTS FOR MEN

Selenium

Selenium is a trace mineral that is essential for good health, having a multitude of functions. It contributes to enzyme function, bone development and helps to transmit nerve impulses. It is found in every cell in the body and shows in the skin, hair and nails. Selenium aids male infertility and is required for prostaglandin production and good hormone balance. This includes the production of healthy sperm in men, as well as trouble-free menstruation and menopause in women. The RDA is 55 mcg.

Brazil nuts are a good source of selenium, so a couple of Brazil nuts every day is beneficial for all, particularly for men. Walnuts, scallops, oysters, free-range eggs and organic vegetables are also good sources of selenium. If taking a supplement, do not exceed the recommended dose, as selenium is toxic in higher quantities.

Vitamin A

Vitamin A is important in sperm formation and helps to prevent DNA damage in sperm. An antioxidant vitamin needed for healthy eyes and skin, it promotes a healthy immune system and is essential for the growth and development of cells. Deficiency in vitamin A affects vision and is also linked to infertility in men. The RDA is 800 mcg. Take care if taking a supplement, however, as an overload of vitamin A causes nausea, vomiting, dizziness, intense headaches, aching joints and tiredness. Foods rich in vitamin A are liver and fish liver oils.

Vitamin C

Vitamin C is necessary for iron absorption, amino acid metabolism, healthy skin and eyes, boosting the immune system and helping to prevent DNA damage in male sperm. The RDA for vitamin C is 80 mg. If you find your iron levels are low, it may help to drink orange juice with an iron-rich meal to increase absorption, or combine iron and vitamin C in a supplement. Vitamin C cannot be stored in the body, so it needs to be replenished daily. See page 193 for a list of dietary sources.

Vitamin E

This antioxidant fights inflammation, helps support cell membranes and prevents deterioration of body fats, particularly the essential fatty acids and other unsaturated fats which, by their nature, are easily damaged. Foods rich in vitamin E include leafy green vegetables, seed oils, cereals, eggs, avocados, sweet potatoes, nuts and seeds, cod liver oil and animal foods. Men need 12 mg per day.

Zinc

Zinc is needed for the formation of healthy bones and teeth, nails, hair and skin. It has antioxidant activity that keeps your immune system strong. Zinc is needed by a developing foetus for formation of the skeleton, growth of the nervous system and brain function.

In men, the prostate gland has one of the highest concentrations of zinc in the body. It is responsible for the production of seminal fluid, in which the sperm swim and are nourished, and is involved in the production of the male hormone testosterone, and has a role in maintaining a healthy libido. Zinc deficiency is associated with a low sperm count and reduced motility.

Men need about 10 mg of zinc per day. Good dietary sources include meat, eggs, green vegetables and seafood, especially oysters (which can contain as much as 50 mg of zinc per 100 g), scallops, prawns, lobster, cockles, mussels and crab.

Watch your weight

Being either underweight or overweight is equally unhelpful when you are trying to conceive. But what is your ideal weight? The chart on page 200 will give you a broad idea of whether your weight falls within the healthy range.

Another way is to calculate your body mass index (BMI). Your BMI will tell you whether your weight is healthy, based on an assessment of your height in relation to your weight. Your BMI can be worked out using a simple calculation:

Your weight in kilograms ÷ (your height in metres)² = BMI

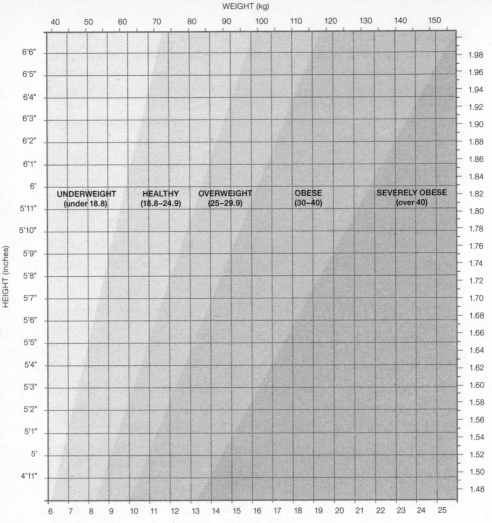

WEIGHT (kg)

40 50 60 70 80 90 100 110 120 130 140 150

HEIGHT (inches)

6'6" 6'5" 6'4" 6'3" 6'2" 6'1" 6' 5'11" 5'10" 5'9" 5'8" 5'7" 5'6" 5'5" 5'4" 5'3" 5'2" 5'1" 5' 4'11"

| UNDERWEIGHT (under 18.8) | HEALTHY (18.8–24.9) | OVERWEIGHT (25–29.9) | OBESE (30–40) | SEVERELY OBESE (over 40) |

HEIGHT (metres)

1.98 1.96 1.94 1.92 1.90 1.88 1.86 1.84 1.82 1.80 1.78 1.76 1.74 1.72 1.70 1.68 1.66 1.64 1.62 1.60 1.58 1.56 1.54 1.52 1.50 1.48

6 7 8 9 10 11 12 13 14 15 16 17 18 19 20 21 22 23 24 25

WEIGHT (stones)

For example, 70kg ÷ (1.7m)^2 = a BMI of 24. According to the World Health Organization, a healthy BMI is between 18.8 and 24.9. You can also calculate your BMI by asking your family doctor or by using one of the many online BMI calculators.

- A BMI of less than 18.8 suggests that you are underweight.
- A BMI of 18.8–24.9 is ideal.
- A BMI of 25–29.9 suggests that you are overweight.
- A BMI of more than 30 is an indicator of obesity.

Eating habits and lifestyle choices have a great impact on your weight. Your health can be readily improved by adjusting the quantities and balance of protein and fruits, vegetables and carbohydrate that are eaten each day. The Chinese ancients said, *'Eat until you are only 70 per cent full – and that should be enough.'*

If your weight is within the healthy range

If your weight is within the healthy range for your height, you should plan to eat three proper meals a day (one of them breakfast) and have healthy snacks of fresh fruit in between meals.

Recommendations I would suggest your diet comprises 25 per cent protein-rich foods, 25 per cent carbohydrate foods and 50 per cent fruits and vegetables.

Aim for three hours of exercise per week. I would recommend that you do whatever kind of exercise you enjoy, as long as it includes some cardiac exercise and stretches as part of a general fitness programme.

If you are underweight

Being underweight reduces your chances of conceiving and increases the possibility of amenorrhea and premature ovarian failure in women and increased numbers of abnormal sperm in men.

Although a small percentage of underweight patients may be underweight as a result of extreme dieting and a desire to look a certain way, the vast majority are desperate to put on weight. No matter how much they eat, nothing changes. I totally understand this situation as many people who are chronically underweight seem to have a faster than average metabolism, which means they burn food quicker than most.

Recommendations I always tease underweight patients and tell them that they are lucky as they can eat whatever they like or as much as they like. If you are underweight, I would recommend that you should eat three BIG meals per day but with no snacks in between.

I would suggest your diet comprises 20 per cent protein-rich foods, 35 per cent carbohydrates and 45 per cent fruit and vegetables. Your diet should also include more unsaturated fats than are usually recommended.

Exercise should be gentle. Try a programme of pilates or yoga, or go swimming. Avoid too much cardiac exercise, which will increase your metabolism and burn off too much body fat.

If you are overweight

Being overweight increases the risk of ovarian malfunction, chromosome abnormality in sperm and eggs, and implantation difficulties. Unfortunately, those who are obese will significantly reduce their chances of conception, and also have an increased risk of diabetes and heart disease.

Recommendations Eating the right kinds of foods improves energy levels and stabilizes mood, staving off tiredness and irritability. If you want to lose weight, regular and frequent small meals are essential to help promote a healthy metabolism.

The proportions of food I would suggest per day are 30 per cent protein-rich foods, 20 per cent carbohydrates and 50 per cent fruit and vegetables. Choose fruit as a snack if you want to eat between meals. Particular attention should be paid to avoiding saturated fats and sugar.

Choose cardiac exercise such as running or working out in the gym. If possible, work with a personal trainer once a week as it will motivate you to work harder and your trainer will encourage you to 'go the extra mile'. Aim for four to five hours of exercise per week.

BEAT SUGAR CRAVINGS

Eating protein is the best way to stave off sugar cravings, as it helps slow the release of sugar in the blood stream and prevents those mid-morning energy dips. Try including some form of protein in your breakfast, such as eggs, bacon, nuts and seeds, smoked salmon or mackerel. Vegetarians should add nuts and seeds to their daily diet, particularly at breakfast time for that early protein boost.

Foods to enjoy, restrict and avoid

A balanced diet includes certain foods that should be eaten often, some just occasionally and a few that should be avoided completely.

FOODS TO ENJOY

In general, the foods that can be eaten with few restrictions are:

- **Fruit** Apples (one a day), bananas and pears (no more than three small portions a week), kiwis, oranges, grapefruits, plums, nectarines, peaches, strawberries, blueberries, apricots, grapes, raspberries, blackberries and watermelon.
- **Vegetables** Spinach, beans, peas, lentils, broccoli, cauliflower, carrots, potatoes, watercress, garlic, onions, leeks, tomatoes, yams, sweet potatoes, lettuce, Brussels sprouts, cabbage, pumpkin and any green vegetables.
- **Protein** I recommend including at least one of the following in each meal: lean meat, organic or free-range chicken, fish, eggs, beans, lentils, nuts and seeds.
- **Fibre** Whole grains, such as wheat, barley, cereals, rice (particularly brown rice), oats and rye; and root vegetables.

FOODS TO BE CAUTIOUS ABOUT

The foods that we should eat less often and in small quantities are:

- **Red meat** Red meat and processed meats like sausages.
- **Dairy products** Cheese, full-fat milk, cream and butter.
- **Refined foods** Any foods that contain added sugar should be kept to a minimum and eaten only occasionally. These include white bread, white pasta and rice, biscuits, chocolate and sweets. White flour causes constipation, which hinders the expulsion of toxins from the body and can reduce fertility. By switching to wholegrain bread and other foods you improve the digestive system function and can therefore improve your fertility.
- **Caffeine** Caffeine intake has been linked to decreased fertility levels, so I would recommend avoiding it completely if possible. If you find that difficult, reduce your consumption of caffeinated drinks to no more than two to three cups a week.

FOODS TO AVOID

Some things should be avoided completely because they offer no nutritional benefit and can be harmful to both the parents' health and that of the developing baby.

- **Smoking** Smoking is not a food as such, but it has been associated with infertility and the early onset of menopause in women, as well as sperm problems in men. It also reduces the success of fertility treatments.
- **Chilled drinks** Drinks with added ice or drinks taken straight from the fridge can irritate your digestive system.
- **Alcohol** Couples who come to see me often ask whether they are allowed a glass of wine with dinner. It is not realistic to expect couples who have been trying to become pregnant for a long time to keep their life on hold and not drink at all.

However, let's understand why some authorities say no to alcohol altogether. Alcohol is a teratogen (a substance known to be harmful to the development of the developing foetus). When a woman's menstrual cycle starts, one or more follicles in her ovaries start to develop. It usually takes 11 to 21 days from the beginning of the cycle for those follicles to mature and release an egg, which could go on to be fertilized. Alcohol could harm the developing foetus from this point on. If fertilization has taken place, alcohol will pass from your blood through the placenta and to your baby, increasing the risk of birth defects and low birth weight.

So, if you do choose to drink, you can protect your possible unborn baby by drinking no more than two small glasses of good-quality wine per week with a meal, or opt for lower alcohol wines and drink plenty of water. Because of the risk to the developing foetus, you should avoid drinking alcohol completely if you know you are pregnant or you are attending assisted fertility treatment.

FOODS FOR SPECIFIC FERTILITY PROBLEMS

You can help improve specific fertility problems by avoiding certain foods and eating more of others.

Polycystic ovaries or Polycystic Ovary Syndrome (PCOS)

Avoid dairy and yeast products wherever possible and switch to soy or other non-dairy products. Keep your carbohydrate intake low. Chilli and hot curry should be off the menu, but do eat foods that are rich in protein.

Endometriosis

Avoid dairy and yeast products. Eat plenty of foods rich in vitamin C, such as fruits and vegetables. High-fibre foods rich in vitamin B can also help reduce the effects of endometriosis on your fertility. Avoid spicy dishes and those ice-cold drinks from the fridge.

Irregular ovulation

Choose foods rich in vitamin B, such as wholegrain cereals, bread, lean red meat, egg yolks, green vegetables, pulses, sweetcorn, brown rice and berries.

Fibroids

Reduce your intake of meat, alcohol and sugar and increase your consumption of fibre. If bleeding is heavy, eat iron-rich foods (lean red meat, sardines and green vegetables) as well as whole grains, or take an iron supplement when necessary.

High prolactin levels

Reduce your intake of protein and increase your consumption of foods rich in vitamin B6, such as oily fish, bananas, lean meat and liver. Vitamin B6 supports the activities of the nervous system and helps to break down sugars and starches.

Healthy eating and TCM

In Traditional Chinese Medicine, all food is considered to have its own character and function which may contribute to your own specific bodily needs. Foods have different flavours and are commonly described as being bitter, sour, salty, sweet and pungent.

Each category affects particular organs of the body.

- **Bitter** foods affect the Heart and Small Intestine. These are cooling foods, sometimes described as 'bitter and drying'. They are used to clear away Heat and dry Damp. They include lettuce, asparagus, cucumber and coffee.
- **Sour** foods affect the Liver and Gall Bladder. These are astringent foods that are used to prevent, absorb or block conditions such as diarrhoea, coughs or perspiration. Citrus fruits such as lemon are classified as sour, as are some sweet fruits such as pears. Tomatoes, olives, mangos, grapes and vinegar also fall into this category.
- **Salty** foods affect the Kidney and Urinary Bladder. Salty foods are considered to soften hardness and lubricate the Intestines to make things descend. Salt, seaweed, some offal and shellfish fall into this category.
- **Sweet** foods affect the Stomach and Spleen. Sweet foods are highly nutritious. They include fruits, grains and many kinds of meat. They are foods that are used to counter-balance the toxic effects of other foods. They nourish, moisten and harmonize. Sweet foods are generally used to treat deficiencies (see pages 211–213).
- **Pungent** foods affect the Lung and Large Intestine. The foods in this category are described as 'dispersing and flowing'. They help to promote the flow of *qi* and also clear toxins from the body. They include herbs and some spices, as well as onions and garlic.

THE *YIN* AND *YANG* OF FOOD

As with everything in Chinese medicine, food categories also affect the *yin–yang* balance. Foods can be divided into: Hot, Cold, Warm and Cool, commonly known as the 'four natures'.

Every food is viewed as having *yin*, *yang* or neutral properties. *Yang* foods are warming, stimulating and dry, whereas *yin* foods are cooling, calming and wet, which may sometimes convert to Damp. Different foods may be added to or eliminated in your diet, depending on your TCM type (see pages 117–136).

Cool–Cold = Yin These foods are used to clear Heat and eliminate toxins.

Warm–Hot = Yang These foods are used to expel Cold and restore *yang*.

There are also various neutral foods that share the characteristics of both.

Warming *yang* foods are eaten more often during the cold months of the year; cooling *yin* foods during the heat of the summer. The warming or cooling effects derive from the nature of the food and the herbs or spices they are cooked with, rather than the temperature at which they are served.

Generally speaking, the sweeter the food, the more *yin* energy it holds. Fruits and vegetables tend to be *yin*. This reflects in cooking methods too: *yin* methods are light, fast and keep the nutrients intact, such as steaming, sautéing and stir-frying.

Yang foods tend more towards the salty and savoury. Meat and animal products such as offal are all *yang* (though fish and eggs are neutral.) *Yang*-style cooking methods include stewing, casseroling, baking and roasting.

CALMING FOODS

Yin

Fruit and vegetables: tofu, celery, melon, grapefruit, watermelon, strawberries, watercress, yellow beans, sprouts, pineapple, pomegranates, cucumber, mushrooms, mangos, pak choi, coriander, lemons, tomatoes, carrots, asparagus, lettuce, cauliflower

Protein-rich foods: cod, lemon sole, sea bass, rabbit, crab, oysters

Drinks: gin, tonic water, white wine

Very *yin*

Fruit and vegetables: bananas, pears, mint, green beans and green bean products, bean sprouts

Neutral

Fruit and vegetables: avocados, chickpeas, apples, peaches, papayas, grapes, plums, cabbage, spinach, onions

Protein-rich foods: chicken, pork, duck, eggs, seeds, nuts, octopus, squid, cuttlefish, clams, eels, lobster, trout, mackerel, dover sole, turbot, lentils

Carbohydrates: brown and white rice, sweet potatoes, oats, bread, coconut, dates, honey.

STIMULATING FOODS

Yang

Fruit and vegetables: garlic, fennel, chives, basil, rosemary, rocket

Protein-rich foods: red beans, black beans, beef, pigeon, pheasant, goose, venison, bacon, ham, liver, kidney, anchovies, tuna, mussels, monkfish, mullet, sardines, prawns

Carbohydrates: roasted nuts, almonds, walnuts, roasted seeds, chips

Spices: black pepper, white pepper, ginger

Drinks: red wine, coffee

Very *yang*

Protein-rich foods: lamb, oxtail

Herbs and spices: ginger, sage, thyme, star anise, cloves, aniseed, cinnamon bark

Drinks: spirits such as whisky, brandy, port

THE HEALING POWER OF TEA

Tea-drinking is a well-established part of Chinese culture and the therapeutic properties of teas are well respected. All true teas come from the plant *Camellia sinesis*. However, there are many different ways of preparing the tea leaves and each part of the leaf is classified according to its quality and brewing qualities.

Green tea The leaves are wilted and crushed. Green tea is not oxidized. It is considered to be extremely health-giving. However, it should not be drunk in large quantities and not all the time. Green tea is very *yin*; it is a cooling tea. If too much is drunk it can cause *yang* deficiency. Green tea is often mixed with other flavours, such as jasmine. Pu erh tea is a matured green tea that has been cured over a longer period of time and is highly sought after.

Black tea The leaves are wilted, sometimes crushed and fully oxidized. Most people in the West are familiar with black tea. It is classified in TCM as warming. Black tea can vary hugely in quality; I usually recommend that patients buy the best-quality tea they can afford and drink it in small quantities. Some of the supermarket teas are slightly *yang* and should be drunk sparingly, though they are good for a *yang*-deficient type. A high-quality black Darjeeling tea such as Earl Grey is neutral and can be drunk more frequently. Black tea is sometimes known as red tea in China, owing to the colour of the liquid once it is brewed (not to be confused with red bush (rooibus) tea).

Oolong tea Wu Long or oolong tea falls somewhere between green tea and black tea. It undergoes a natural drying and fermenting process and is high in polyphenols, which are present in antioxidants. It is particularly good for the digestion and is said to reduce high blood pressure.

Rooibos (Red bush) Rooibos comes from South Africa. It is a neutral tea made from the oxidized leaves of the plant *Aspalanthus linearis*. It can be drunk at any time, especially if taken without milk. It is caffeine free.

White tea White tea is rarer than the other teas. It is made from the buds of the white peony plant and is the least oxidized of all the teas. It is good for *yin* types and those who have lost Heat.

Others Herb teas, fruit teas and flower teas each have their own properties and are caffeine free. Some are warming, some are cooling. It is best not to drink any tea to the exclusion of all others. Variety is important. I usually recommend that a tea bag should be reused so that the dilution is weak and a single bag lasts a whole day.

Eating for your TCM type

Depending on which TCM categories you fall into, you might like to try eating more or less of the following foods. It is important to eat a wide variety of foods. My recommendation to achieve a balanced diet is buy only the foods from the *Foods to eat* lists below. Save the *Foods to avoid* as treats for special occasions, perhaps when you are dining out.

BLOOD STASIS

Blood stasis in a woman's reproductive system is a common result of *qi* stagnation, prolonged Cold exposure, Phlegm-Damp or Damp-Heat. Eating the proper foods can help prevent the condition getting worse, but it is only a partial solution.

Foods to eat: For those who have been diagnosed as having Blood stasis, iron-rich and high-fibre foods can help. A small glass of red wine can be drunk, but remember not to exceed more than two to three glasses per week.

Herbs and spices: garlic, nutmeg, chives, parsley

Vegetables, fruit and nuts: aubergine, leafy greens, leeks, onions, beetroot, seaweeds, spinach, figs, apricots, cherries, blackberries, dates, grapes, lychees, peaches, strawberries, chestnuts

Carbohydrates: wholegrain breads and cereals, brown rice, wholewheat pasta, barley, potatoes, root vegetables

Protein-rich foods: bone marrow, lean beef, chicken, eggs, liver, mussels, octopus, squid, sardines, black beans

Others: brown sugar, vinegar

Foods to avoid: When there is a pattern of combined Heat, or *yin* or Blood deficiency, it is important to avoid pungent and Hot foods such as ginger, cinnamon and alcohol.

LIVER QI STAGNATION

It is important to ensure that *qi* moves smoothly and freely around the body, particularly if life and work are stressful and emotions are running high. These are feelings that may prevent the body from adapting quickly enough and *qi* stagnation can result. If this is your type, eat small amounts of easily digestible foods, and increase your levels of movement and relaxation.

Foods to eat: The following foods may help to get *qi* moving again.

Herbs and spices: basil, cardamom, rosemary, chives, garlic, coriander, dill seed, mint, peppermint tea (just one tea bag per day)

Vegetables, fruit and nuts: aubergine, broccoli, carrots, Brussels sprouts, celery, fennel, garlic, leeks, lettuce, onions, radishes, spinach, grapefruit, peaches, plums, lemons, oranges, citrus peel such as orange or tangerine (which can be used as a flavouring in cooking)

Carbohydrates: barley, basmati rice, other rices, rye

Protein-rich foods: chicken, eggs, crab, prawns

Others: vinegar

Foods to avoid: If Liver *qi* stagnation is combined with excessive Heat, avoid horseradish, pepper and prawns.

PHLEGM-DAMP

Phlegm-Damp is often directly related to dietary habits. It can result from unhealthy eating with a preference for rich, sweet foods and too much meat or alcohol.

Foods to eat: Eat drying, bitter-Warm foods.

Herbs and spices: coriander, peppermint, thyme, black pepper, ginger, cinnamon, garlic, cardamom, nutmeg

Vegetables, fruit and nuts: apples, broad beans, citrus peel such as lemon, orange or tangerine, grapefruit, olives, leeks, onions, peppers, squash, plums, grapes, radishes, watercress, almonds, walnuts

Carbohydrates: barley, corn, oats, rice, whole grains, rye, millet

Protein-rich foods: mackerel, sardines, prawns, small amounts of chicken and turkey

Others: lemon and ginger tea (just one tea bag per day), Earl Grey or rooibos (red bush) tea

Foods to avoid: If you have too much Damp in the body, avoid fatty, oily or greasy foods and mucus-producing foods such as dairy products. Cut back on sweet foods and sugar in all forms, especially chocolate. Also avoid wheat and yeast-based foods such as bread and cakes, and fatty meats like pork.

DAMP-HEAT
Accumulations of Damp and Heat are also related to the diet, so the recommendations are similar to those for Phlegm-Damp. Damp-Heat can result from a poor diet of greasy and sweet foods, too much meat and too much alcohol.

Foods to eat: Increase levels of bitter-cool foods.

Herbs and spices: cardamom, basil, mint

Vegetables, fruit and nuts: aubergine, bean sprouts, broad beans, broccoli, cabbage, celery, cucumber, lettuce, onions, seaweed, water chestnuts, watercress, dandelion leaves, apples, bananas, grapefruit, grapes, lemons, pears, tomatoes

Carbohydrates: corn, rice, rye, barley

Protein-rich foods: anchovies, black soya beans, mackerel, sardines, snails, tofu, mung beans, kidney beans, small amounts of chicken and turkey

Others: horseradish, salt, elderflower, green tea, jasmine tea (just one tea bag or one small teaspoonful of loose tea per day)

Foods to avoid: The recommendations are the same as for Phlegm-Damp above.

DRINKING HERBAL TEAS
If you use herbal tea bags, such as lemon and ginger or apple and cinnamon, make one tea bag (or no more than two) last the whole day. A fresh bag steeped in boiling water for several minutes can be too strong for your system. Instead it is good idea to dip the tea bag into the hot water, then take it out quickly and keep it to reuse again later that day, which will avoid overload.

BLOOD HEAT
Too much Heat in the body is *yang* in nature, which harms and dries out *yin*, Blood and body fluids, as well as disrupting peace of mind. Choose cooling, moistening foods to clear Heat and replenish body fluids. People with excess Heat like drinking mint tea – but keep it weak and try to use fresh mint rather than a tea bag.

Foods to eat: Be sure to eat plenty of raw vegetables and salads.

Herbs and spices: mint, peppermint

Vegetables, fruit and nuts: asparagus, carrots, cucumber, celery, lettuce, bananas, lemons, pears, apples, kiwi fruits, pineapple, mangos, tomatoes, watermelon

Carbohydrates: Most types of carbohydrate are good for this type, but avoid toasting and frying.

Protein-rich foods: tofu

Others: elderflower, green tea (use only one tea bag per day), jasmine tea, peppermint tea

Foods to avoid: Try to cut out coffee and alcohol altogether, particularly spirits, and spicy foods such as chilli and curry.

COLD IN THE UTERUS
Cold is *yin* in character and results from external exposure to cold or excessive consumption of cold, raw foods.

Foods to eat: Eat plenty of warming foods such as meat and pungent spices. Try to have soups and herbal teas.

Herbs and spices: black pepper, star anise, coriander, cardamom, cinnamon, cloves, garlic, ginger, mustard, nutmeg, basil, dill, chives, thyme

Vegetables, fruit and nuts: fennel, onions, dates, cherries, lychees, roasted nuts such as cashews and almonds

Carbohydrates: root vegetables such as parsnips, brown rice, whole grains, toast

Protein-rich foods: beef, chicken, lamb, game, prawns, trout, mussels

Others: capers, red wine, whisky

Foods to avoid: Cooling foods such as raw foods and salads. Never eat or drink food straight from the fridge.

QI DEFICIENCY
Qi deficiency generally results from exhaustion, lack of sleep, chronic illness, negative emotions, such as worry, or poor eating habits. Those with *qi* deficiency should eat warming, easy-to-digest foods that help promote *qi*, rebalance the Spleen, build energy and stimulate the metabolism. Note that microwave cooking may reduce the value of the *qi* in food, so adopt other cooking methods where possible.

Foods to eat: Iron- and protein-rich foods such as meat and pulses are key blood-nourishing foods.

Herbs and spices: cardamom, cloves, garlic, ginger, turmeric, sage

Vegetables, fruit and nuts: sweet potatoes, wild mushrooms, figs, dates, cherries, apples, almonds, coconut, cabbage, squash, papayas, aubergine

Carbohydrates: rice, oats, millet

Protein-rich foods: chicken, lean meat, eggs, oily fish such as mackerel and sardines, chickpeas

Foods to avoid: Hot, bitter and acidic foods such as spices or alcohol should be avoided. Try also to avoid sugar and dairy products like full-fat milk, cheese and butter.

BLOOD DEFICIENCY

Choose moistening and nourishing foods to supplement the Blood. Protein-rich foods are beneficial and whole grains have a particularly nourishing effect.

Foods to eat: Iron-rich and high-fibre foods can help with Blood deficiency.

Herbs and spices: sage, chives

Vegetables, fruit and nuts: dark leafy greens, spinach, seaweeds, broccoli, dates, figs, blackberries, beetroot, cherries, strawberries, almonds, cashew nuts, coconut

Carbohydrates: rice, oats, root vegetables such as sweet potatoes and yams

Protein-rich foods: squid, octopus, liver, sardines, herring, mackerel, black beans, lentils, eggs, lean red meat, game

Others: milk

Foods to avoid: Avoid pungent and Hot foods that dry fluids and Blood, like curry spices, ginger, chilli and alcohol, especially when there is a pattern of combined Heat.

KIDNEY *YIN* DEFICIENCY

Yin foods are moist, cooling foods that have a soothing effect on the body (see pages 205–206).

Foods to eat: Eat plenty of fresh fruit and vegetables. Leafy green vegetables are especially beneficial.

Herbs and spices: fresh basil, chives, coriander, parsley; small amounts of garlic or ginger

Vegetables, fruit and nuts: asparagus, avocados, peas, cabbage, seaweeds, spinach, spring onions, carrots, pumpkin, apples, lemons, tomatoes, bananas, oranges, mangos, raspberries, pineapple, pomegranates, almonds, sesame seeds, sunflower seeds, walnuts

Carbohydrates: millet, wheat, rice, spelt, potatoes, sweet potatoes, yams

Protein-rich foods: bone marrow, chicken, crab, duck, eggs, sardines, mussels, kidneys, lobster, liver, mussels, oysters, pork, goose, rabbit, snails, tofu, lentils, mung beans, kidney beans

Others: honey, skimmed or semi-skimmed milk, miso, olive oil

Foods to avoid: Avoid warming foods such as cloves, cinnamon, thyme, chilli, curry spices and pepper. Eat red meat only occasionally.

KIDNEY *YANG* DEFICIENCY

Yang foods warm and invigorate the body. Nutritional therapy involves boosting the Spleen *qi* and Kidney *yang*.

Foods to eat: Include warming foods in your diet, such as spices, lean meats and easily digestible grains.

Herbs and spices: aniseed, basil, cumin, black pepper, chives, cinnamon bark, cloves, ginger, rocket, mustard, rosemary, sage, star anise, thyme, white pepper, garlic, parsley, nutmeg, oregano, juniper berries, cardamom

Vegetables, fruit and nuts: fennel, onions, leeks, parsnips, turnips, apples, apricots, plums, roasted almonds, roasted seeds, walnuts

Carbohydrates: buckwheat, brown rice, potatoes, oats, spelt, quinoa

Protein-rich foods: black beans and other pulses, beef, beef broth, venison, chicken, lamb, oxtail, game, anchovies, liver, kidneys, tuna, mussels, monkfish, mullet, sardines, prawns, salmon, trout, bacon, ham

Others: coffee, whisky, brandy, red wine in limited amounts

Foods to avoid: Avoid cold drinks and foods eaten straight from the fridge. Some fruits, such as watermelon, bananas, cranberries and pears, slow down the movement of fluids in the body so try to avoid these.

Simple healthy recipes

Eating well improves your general health and can also have a positive effect on your reproductive health. A sustaining and nutritional breakfast at the start of the day is particularly important. After a long period of rest without food overnight, the metabolism slows down, so a kick-start will help your body and your brain to wake up and function properly again. The body is like a machine: it needs to be programmed, so don't skip breakfast, just set aside 10 minutes for it every day. It is very important, particularly when you're trying to get pregnant.

SIMPLE BREAKFASTS

The following breakfasts are easy to digest and very warming, ideal to improve your body's metabolism.

- **Baked beans on toast** Choose wholegrain brown bread and low-sugar baked beans.
- **Egg on toast** Choose wholegrain brown bread for toasting and serve with a poached or boiled egg.
- **Bacon and toast** Choose wholegrain brown bread served with lean bacon that has been grilled, not fried.
- **Cereal** Choose a good-quality wholegrain breakfast cereal fortified with minerals and vitamins.
- **Porridge** Oats contain slow-release carbohydrates to keep your blood sugar levels stable, and so control your appetite, until lunch time. Sprinkle with sunflower seeds for a boost of protein and omega-3. See the recipe below.

Porridge

1 cup whole porridge oats
1¼ cups semi-skimmed, skimmed or soya milk
1¼ cups water
handful of mixed seeds or nuts, such as sunflower seeds, pumpkin seeds or almonds
honey, to taste (optional)

- Use a cup or small glass to measure the oats, milk and water. The proportions should be 1 measure of oats to 2½ measures of liquid. Place them in a heavy-based saucepan.
- Bring slowly to the boil, then reduce the heat and simmer gently for 3–5 minutes, depending on the size of the oats used.
- Serve sprinkled with seeds or nuts and drizzled with honey, if liked.

Easy Steamed Chicken

This is a great dish for any time of year. Reserve the bones from the chicken to make a nourishing chicken stock (see below).

1.25 kg (2½ lb) organic free-range chicken
1 tablespoon salt
3 coriander stalks, chopped
1 teaspoon sesame seeds
5 slices of fresh root ginger
1 spring onion, chopped
2 mild red or green chillies, finely sliced
2 tablespoons light soy sauce

Serves 4–6

- Rinse the chicken, pat dry with kitchen paper and sprinkle with the salt, inside and outside. Cover and leave to marinate in the refrigerator overnight.
- Place the chicken in a heatproof dish that fits into a steamer and cook over a saucepan of rapidly simmering water, breast down, for 30 minutes or until cooked through (the juices should run clear when the thickest part of the thigh is pierced with a knife). Leave the chicken in the steamer until it is cool enough to handle.
- Remove the chicken from the dish, reserving the juices. Tear the meat off the bones with your fingers and put into a large bowl. Set the bones to one side to make chicken stock (see below). Drizzle the juices over the meat.
- Add all the other ingredients and toss gently with the chicken. Serve warm or cold, on its own or with salad.

Chicken Stock

High in nutritional value, this stock is rich in protein and calcium because the bones are boiled. The stock can be used to make pasta, rice or noodle dishes, or soups like the one on page 216.

- To make stock out of chicken bones, bring 1 litre (1¾ pints) water to the boil in a large saucepan. Add the chicken bones from a 1.25 kg (2½ lb) organic free-range chicken, and 1 slice of fresh root ginger.
- Bring back to the boil, then reduce the heat and simmer for at least 2 hours. Leave to cool, then strain the stock. This can be served on its own as a broth, or used in cooking. If not used immediately, freeze for later use.

Ping's Chicken Soup

Use the stock made from the chicken bones in the recipe on page 215 to create this delicious soup.

100 g (3½ oz) new potatoes
2 tablespoons sunflower oil
1 white onion, finely sliced
50 g (2 oz) leeks, trimmed, cleaned and chopped
1 garlic clove
750 ml (1¼ pints) chicken stock
100 g (3½ oz) baby spinach
sea salt and freshly ground black pepper

Serves 1–2

- Cook the potatoes in a large saucepan of lightly salted boiling water until tender. Drain, leave to cool, then peel and cut into dice.
- Heat the sunflower oil in a large saucepan and gently cook the onion for 2 minutes. Add the potatoes and leeks and continue to cook until the vegetables are tender.
- Add the garlic and fry gently for about 1 minute, then add the stock. Bring to the boil, then reduce the heat and simmer for 15 minutes.
- Remove from the heat, add the spinach and use a hand-held electric blender to purée the soup until smooth. Season to taste and serve hot.

Lightly Boiled Pak Choi

This pak choi retains its colour during cooking as it is coated with oil to maximize freshness and levels of vitamin C and vitamin E. This method also works well with green beans, but cook for a little longer, about 2 minutes.

500 ml (17 fl oz) water
½ teaspoon sunflower oil
250 g (8 oz) pak choi

Serves 1–2

- Bring the measurement water to the boil in a large saucepan, add the oil and the pak choi and cook for 1 minute.
- Drain the pak choi and serve immediately.

Stir-Fried Beef with Egg and Tomato

This recipe is rich in vitamin C, vitamin D, vitamin B12 and iron. It is also a good source of calcium and protein.

150 g (5 oz) lean beef, thinly sliced
2 tablespoons sunflower oil
450 g (14½ oz) tomatoes, each cut into 6 or 8
100 ml (3½ fl oz) water
1 tablespoon tomato ketchup
2 eggs, lightly beaten
2 spring onions, chopped
1 teaspoon cornflour, mixed with 2 tablespoons water

Seasoning (1)
½ tablespoon light soy sauce
½ teaspoon brown sugar
1 teaspoon cornflour
½ tablespoon water

Seasoning (2)
½ teaspoon salt
1 teaspoon brown sugar
1 teaspoon Thai fish sauce or light soy sauce

Serves 1–2

- Mix the ingredients for Seasoning (1) in a shallow dish, add the beef and leave to marinate for 15 minutes.
- Heat the sunflower oil in a wok or large frying pan and stir-fry the beef for 2–3 minutes or until cooked to your liking. Remove from the pan, set aside and keep warm.
- Add the tomatoes to the pan with the measurement water and bring to the boil, then reduce the heat and simmer gently for 5 minutes. Add the tomato ketchup and Seasoning (2) and mix well.
- Pour the beaten egg into the pan and continue to cook without stirring or covering the pan until the egg is set. Return the beef to the pan with the spring onions, mix well, then stir in the cornflour and water mixture. Heat gently until the sauce thickens, then serve hot.

Stir-Fried Chicken with Vegetables

This combination of chicken and green vegetables packs a nutritional punch in the form of protein, vitamin B2, vitamin C, vitamin E and vitamin K. It is an excellent choice in everyday cooking.

150 g (5 oz) chicken breast fillet, thickly sliced
250 g (8 oz) fine green beans or broccoli, cut into bite-sized pieces
4 teaspoons sunflower oil
1 garlic clove, crushed
½ tablespoon very finely chopped shallot
1 teaspoon rice wine or light cream sherry
100 g (3½ oz) button mushrooms, sliced
2½ teaspoons cornflour, mixed with 2 tablespoons water

Seasoning (1)
¼ teaspoon salt
½ tablespoon cornflour
1 tablespoon oil

Seasoning (2)
dash of sesame oil
pinch of ground white pepper
¼ teaspoon salt
¼ teaspoon brown sugar
½ tablespoon Thai fish sauce or light soy sauce
125 ml (4 fl oz) chicken stock

Serves 1–2

- Mix the ingredients for Seasoning (1) in a shallow dish, add the chicken and leave to marinate for 20 minutes.
- Bring a small saucepan of water to the boil, add the beans or broccoli with 1 teaspoon of the oil and cook for 1 minute. Drain and set aside.
- Heat the remaining oil in a wok or large frying pan, add the garlic and shallot and cook for 1 minute. Add the chicken, stir well and cook until golden, then add the rice wine or sherry and continue stir-frying until cooked through.
- Return the beans or broccoli to the pan with the mushrooms and Seasoning (2) and cook for a further 2 minutes. Add the cornflour and water mixture, heat gently until the sauce thickens, then serve hot.

10 WAYS TO IMPROVE YOUR CHANCES OF CONCEIVING

If you and your partner take an honest look at your lifestyle and are prepared to make some positive changes, you can dramatically increase your chances of conceiving.

1. **Watch what you eat every day** To maximize your chances of getting pregnant, it's important to eat a healthy, balanced diet.

2. **Watch your weight** If you are overweight or very underweight, you are less likely to be able to conceive easily. If you or your partner are obese, consult your doctor for advice on the best and safest way to lose weight gradually.

3. **Be active** Regular, moderate exercise of around 30 minutes a day will help to improve your fitness and keep you at a good weight. It will also boost your endorphin levels, the body's own 'happy hormones'.

4. **Drink wisely** Women who are trying to conceive are advised to avoid alcohol completely. Men should drink no more than two or three small glasses of wine per week.

5. **Don't smoke** Smoking has been associated with infertility and early menopause in women, as well as sperm problems in men. It also reduces the success of fertility treatments.

6. **Keep cool** For optimum sperm production, the testicles should be a couple of degrees cooler than the rest of the body. Men should avoid tight underwear and jeans, cycling and excessively hot baths and saunas. We also recommend showering the testicles with cool water for a few seconds each day.

7. **Take care at work** Occupations that involve sitting for long periods or exposure to environmental chemicals may affect general health in women and may additionally affect sperm quality in men.

8. **Manage stress** We all have different stress thresholds and there is now growing evidence that being stressed can affect your chances of conceiving. The body interprets physiological stressors, such as lack of sleep and intensive athletic training, in the same way as psychological stress caused by excessive anxiety, bereavement or divorce, for example. The stress can sometimes upset your mental health and can disturb your normal bodily functions. So try to identify and reduce the things that cause you stress.

9. **Take folic acid** All women trying for a baby should take a supplement of folic acid every day (see page 193).

10. **Check the side effects of drugs** Certain prescription drugs can reduce the chances of conception, so make sure your doctor is aware that you're trying for a baby.

Chapter 10
ACUPRESSURE AND EXERCISE

Traditionally, Chinese medicine includes a combination of herbal medicine, acupuncture and bodywork, exercise techniques such as Qi Gong or Tai Chi, and therapies such as acupressure, massage, reflexology and moxibustion. These different elements work together to improve health and wellbeing. You obviously need to consult an experienced practitioner of TCM for herbal treatments and acupuncture, but there is much you can do yourself at home to optimize your body's health.

Using self-help methods to keep the body healthy is a wonderful addition to TCM treatment. Techniques such as acupressure and the habit of taking regular exercise will also help to improve the flow of *qi* energy around the body and gently ensure that you are improving your physical condition. A healthy and well-nourished body has a much better chance of healthy egg implantation (provided there are not more serious medical causes).

Exercise and TCM

For a healthy existence, we need a good night's sleep, good nutrition and regular, moderate exercise. Normal physical activity is beneficial to the smooth and healthy running of the human body; it can increase physical strength and prevent illness. However, excessive activity can overwork and weaken the body's constitution.

Regular and moderate exercise increases your oxygen intake which, in turn, improves your circulation, respiration and muscle condition. Exercise also stimulates your brain's chemical reactions powerfully enough to change the way you feel, helping combat anxiety or depression and improve concentration. I wouldn't like to say that exercise alone will necessarily clear any underlying health conditions, but it certainly helps enormously in many cases; and regular exercise is a preventative measure.

Appropriate levels of exercise will:

- Boost your energy levels
- Help relieve stress
- Help maintain better blood sugar levels
- Improve your muscle coordination
- Reduce low-density lipids (bad cholesterol) and increase high-density lipids (good cholesterol)
- Improve your muscle tone
- Make you more flexible and relaxed
- Stimulate hormones, including the sex hormones
- Improve your self-esteem
- Increase your social interaction
- Enhance your self-control, self-confidence and self-discipline

Some people say to me, 'I live a very healthy lifestyle. I don't eat or drink bad things – what have I done wrong? Why can't I get pregnant?' At the end of the day, not everything is related to diet and exercise, and as I have explained before there are many underlying causes that can contribute to your fertility problems. However, keeping your body fit and healthy will always enhance your chances and ensure you are giving yourself the best possible opportunity.

In this section, my exercise advice is simple:

Healthy diet + Exercise = Improved health and wellbeing
That's it.

WHAT TYPE OF EXERCISE?

Practices such as Qi Gong and Tai Chi generally involve slow movements that need concentration. They are very peaceful and meditative. Like yoga, they can be excellent ways to control your breath, or slow you down if you have a tendency to be over-energetic. These practices work the whole body and focus the mind. They are also excellent forms of exercise for people who lead quite sedentary lives or are recovering from illness.

I grew up in China and have practised both Qi Gong and Tai Chi in the past. However, I do not believe that it is essential to learn Chinese exercise systems in order to maintain your health and so I will not insist that you join your local Tai Chi class – unless you want to. We are all different. Some people enjoy energetic sports, others require more gentle activities. The style of exercise you choose will depend on your weight, your energy levels, the time you have available and your body's needs. Most important of all is to do what exercise you enjoy most so you will be motivated to keep doing it on a regular basis.

I always say to patients that they need to take into account what they really enjoy, so they will be better able to keep it up. My own preference is to play tennis. It gives me an excellent cardiovascular workout and improves flexibility. It is also mentally stimulating, it is sociable and it pushes me to stretch myself that little bit harder because it is competitive. But if you have a lot of weight to lose and you are not used to exercising, you may prefer to start slowly, with less intensive exercise such as walking and a yoga class, until your energy levels and motivation have increased.

Getting started

Fitness levels take time to build up. It is not unusual for someone to find themselves out of breath when running on a treadmill for ten minutes; but it is remarkable how well the body can improve if you take things slowly. It won't take long before ten minutes on the treadmill feels less strenuous.

EXERCISE HINTS AND TIPS

- Do something every day.
- Make sure it is something you enjoy.
- Whatever you do, ensure you increase your oxygen intake by taking deep breaths and then completely exhaling – that is, increasing the length of your exhale.
- Do not overexert yourself, but do make sure that you exercise sufficiently to raise your heart rate for at least 20 minutes (enough to raise a sweat) three to five times a week.

HOW MUCH EXERCISE?

I am often asked how much exercise is enough and how much is too much. It is unwise to be too prescriptive about this; instead I say to people, listen to your body and pay attention to how you feel. That said, it is true that if you are overweight or classified as obese in medical terms, the statistical results suggest that your body may find it harder to conceive. If you haven't exercised for some time, it is very important to begin slowly and with the guidance of your family doctor.

Refer to the weight chart on page 200 to see whether you need to lose weight or whether you are in the healthy weight range.

- If you are underweight, choose low cardiac activities, so you don't burn off too many calories when exercising.
- If you are average to slightly overweight, aim to exercise for two or three hours a week (that's 20 to 30 minutes a day).
- If you are overweight, plan to exercise for four or five hours a week (that's 40 to 45 minutes a day).

If, after exercise, you feel energized and great, that means you are doing the right amount for you. If you are not tired or sweating and do not feel energized, you are not doing enough for your needs. If you feel exhausted or overtired, then you are doing too much.

GETTING HELP

I would always recommend that, if you can afford it, it is worth having a personal trainer who can help to tailor a programme to your needs. They will also either encourage you to push yourself harder, or suggest you take things at a more steady pace, depending on your progress. There are gym instructors and qualified trainers at every gym or sports club, so ask for help and make sure that you are monitoring your progress and adapting your programme in line with your needs.

KEEPING ON THE MOVE

Exercising in an appropriate way can balance your physical and mental health. Obviously, different types of exercise have different benefits, so you should think about the result you're looking for, then choose the most appropriate exercise.

A moderate exercise regime could be one of the following:
Outdoor running: 15 to 20 minutes, three times a week
Walking: a brisk walk of 20 to 30 minutes a day
Gym exercise: 40 to 45 minutes, two or three times a week
Swimming: 20 to 30 minutes, three times a week

For gentle weight loss, choose one of these:
Pilates or yoga: one hour, twice a week
Swimming: 10 to 15 minutes, two or three times a week
Walking: a brisk walk of 20 to 30 minutes a day

For greater weight loss, choose one of these:
Outdoor running: 30 to 40 minutes, three times a week
Gym exercise: one hour, three times a week
Swimming: 30 to 40 minutes, three times a week

Keep your arms and legs moving correctly while you exercise so that you encourage improved blood circulation. The muscles of the arms and legs act as pumps to assist the working of the heart, encouraging the flow of blood and lymph around the body. Lymph is a colourless liquid which delivers oxygen and nutrients to the tissues via the blood stream, while also removing waste products. The lymphatic system has no pump of its own, so it is completely dependent on regular and effective muscular activity.

Acupressure and fertility

Acupressure, like acupuncture, focuses on key points along the meridians of the body (see pages 38–52) to encourage the flow of *qi* and release blockages. The difference is that you can do it to yourself, no matter where you are. The system is over 3,000 years old and is used not only to maintain general health and wellbeing, but also as a method of pain relief.

Like acupuncture, acupressure is used to balance the body by either clearing blockages or stimulating the flow of Blood and *qi*. It can be used to help improve fertility problems and is invaluable in aiding relaxation when you are trying to conceive. Stress-related conditions such as headaches, feelings of nausea and low energy can be readily treated with acupressure.

Acupressure involves applying pressure on specific points on the meridians of the body, using the fingertips or thumb (whichever is more comfortable) to either reduce or tonify the activity of the organs. This can be done by tapping, or by applying deeper pressure, depending on what you feel you need and where on the body you need to apply the pressure.

The location of each acupressure point is measured in cun.

- **1 cun** = the thickness of the thumb at the knuckle.
- **1.5 cun** = the width of two forefingers.
- **3 cun** = the width of all four fingers, side by side.

Once you have located the relevant point, use your fingers or thumb to work the point for two to three minutes. That should be long enough to make a difference. You can always reapply the pressure again later. The point shouldn't hurt, but it may feel a bit numb or may ache when the pressure is applied. You may find your fingers ache a little, too. You can really only work on those points that you can see or reach, so the guidelines that follow are all based on self-help.

WARNING

Some of the acupressure points used to aid fertility are the same as those used to induce birth during late pregnancy. They may therefore contribute to the chances of miscarriage if used during pregnancy. It is advisable to STOP USING ACUPRESSURE ONCE YOU BECOME PREGNANT, unless you are being guided by a qualified TCM practitioner, to avoid any confusion over which points should be used and which not.

CONCEPTION VESSEL

See page 51 for a full description of the Conception Vessel. The following points are those commonly used in acupressure.

CV-4 *Guan Yuan* (Gateway to Original *Qi*)

This point is located 3 cun below the navel. It is used to tonify vital energy, particularly *qi* and Blood deficiencies. This point is great for both men and women. It is also useful for treating genito-urinary conditions such as incontinence.

In the case of fertility problems, it can be used for menstrual disorders where there are deficiencies, Cold or stagnation present – such as amenorrhea or pale blood. In men, it can be useful for treating impotence.

CV-6 *Qi Hai* (Sea of *Qi*)

This point is located 1.5 cun below the navel and 1 cun above CV-4. It is used generally for tonifying *qi*. In women it is used for treating tiredness, irregular menstruation, period pains or cramps and amenorrhea. In men it is useful for treating symptoms of impotence and night-time urination.

GOVERNING VESSEL

See page 52 for a full description of the Governing Vessel. The following point is the one commonly used in acupressure.

GV-3 *Yao Yang Guan* (Barrier of the *Yang*)

This point is located at the base of the spine in the gap between the fourth and fifth lumbar vertebra. It is used to treat lower back pain from Kidney deficiency, painful periods, irregular menstruation, impotence, incontinence and fertility-related problems.

STOMACH MERIDIAN

See page 41 for a full description of the Stomach Meridian. The following points are those commonly used in acupressure.

ST-25 *Tian Shu* (Heaven's Pivot)

This point can be found 2 cun either side of the belly button. It has a powerful effect on the Large Intestine and is commonly used to ease constipation, stomach pain or diarrhoea. Importantly, it is also useful in treating menstrual problems, fibroids and other blockages related to fertility issues.

ST-28 *Shui Dao* (Waterway)

This point can be found 3 cun below ST-25. It is used to treat excess Cold and *qi* and Blood stagnation resulting in painful periods, fibroids, cysts and other fertility issues in women that are related to Cold obstructing the uterus.

Caution: DO NOT USE THIS POINT WHEN YOU ARE PREGNANT.

ST-29 *Gui Lai* **(Return)**

This point can be found 4 cun below ST-25. It is used in the treatment of *qi* stagnation, irregular menstruation, amenorrhoea, period pains, vaginal discharge and Cold in the uterus. In men it is used to treat genital pain or swelling, and impotence.

Caution: DO NOT USE THIS POINT WHEN YOU ARE PREGNANT.

ST-36 *Zu San Li* **(Leg Three Miles)**

This is a very important point for building and maintaining overall health. It is located 3 cun below the knee and is used to tonify deficient *qi* or Blood and is a very important point for building and maintaining overall health. It is used to treat all conditions connected with the Stomach or the Spleen, including premenstrual tension, bloating, nausea, vomiting, hiccups, constipation, diarrhoea, as well as breast problems, lower leg pain, depression, fatigue and nervousness. It is also known to improve the immune system. Five minutes is enough time to work this point.

SPLEEN MERIDIAN

See page 42 for a full description of the Spleen Meridian. The following points are those commonly used in acupressure.

SP-6 *San Yin Jiao* **(Three *Yin* Intersection)**

This point can be found 3 cun above the top of the ankle on the inside of the leg and just behind the tibia leg bone. It marks the intersection of three different meridians – Spleen, Liver and Kidney – so it has quite a powerful impact and is very good for blood circulation. It is used to tonify *yin* and Blood. In fertility treatment, this point is used when a patient is suffering from insomnia, palpitations and other anxiety-related emotions, as well as irregular, stopped and painful periods. It is also used to treat male sexual issues.

Caution: DO NOT USE THIS POINT WHEN YOU ARE PREGNANT as it is also used for inducing labour.

SP-9 *Yin Ling Quan* **(*Yin* Mound Spring)**

This point can be found in the hollow below the knee, near the tibia. If you feel sensitivity here it indicates a blockage. By working the point you will help to relieve it. SP-9 regulates the Spleen, transforms Dampness stagnation, clears Damp-Heat (especially from the genitals) and aids with menstrual problems, oedema and urinary problems such as incontinence.

SP-10 *Xue Hai* **(Sea of Blood)**

This point is located 2 cun above the knee cap and 1 cun to the inside of the leg above SP-9. It is used to treat Heat in the Blood, irregular menstruation, painful and heavy periods, rashes, eczema and abdominal distension; or when there is a lot of Heat in the body.

Caution: USE ONLY UNDER SUPERVISION FROM A TCM PRACTITIONER.

URINARY BLADDER MERIDIAN

See page 45 for a full description of the Urinary Bladder Meridian. The following points are those commonly used in acupressure.

UB-18 *Gan Shu* (Liver *Shu*)
This point is good for balancing Liver function to help build menstrual blood, reduce stress and relax the muscles. It is found 1.5 cun either side of the spine, level with the base of the ninth thoracic vertebra.

UB-20 *Pi Shu* (Spleen *Shu*)
This point is good for helping to clear Damp and Phlegm, and acts to tonify the digestive function. It is found 1.5 cun either side of the spine, level with the eleventh thoracic vertebra.

UB-23 *Shen Shu* (Kidney *Shu*)
This point is good for backache and fatigue. It also acts to tonify the Kidney function to help the reproductive system as a whole. It is found 1.5 cun either side of the spine, level with the space between the second and third lumbar vertebrae.

UB-25 *Dachang Shu* (Large Intestine *Shu*)
This point is good for treating tiredness due to too much Damp and Phlegm. It is found 1.5 cun either side of the spine, level with base of the fourth lumbar vertebra.

UB-31 *Shang Liao* (Upper Crevice),
UB-32 *Ci Liao* (Second Crevice),
UB-33 *Zhong Liao* (Middle Crevice),
UB-34 *Xia Liao* (Lower Crevice)

These points tend to be considered together because their function is similar. Located on the lower back, these points, when massaged, promote bladder function and are helpful for improving fertility. The back is quite difficult to reach, so try buying a massage cushion and placing on those areas for the same effect.

Caution: DO NOT USE THESE FOUR POINTS WHEN YOU ARE PREGNANT as they are also used for inducing labour.

LARGE INTESTINE MERIDIAN
See page 40 for a full description of the Large Intestine Meridian. The following point is commonly used in acupressure.

LI-4 *He Gu* (Joining Valley)
This point is easily located on the back of your hand in the soft tissue between thumb and first finger. It relieves pain from headaches and tension and is also very effective for easing period pain. It is generally used with CV-4 for tonifying *qi*.

Caution: DO NOT USE THIS POINT WHEN YOU ARE PREGNANT as it is also used for inducing labour.

PERICARDIUM MERIDIAN

See page 47 for a full description of the Pericardium Meridian. The following point is commonly used in acupressure.

PC-6 *Nei Guan* (Inner Pass)

This point is located 2 cun above the crease of the wrist. It is an excellent calming point and is also great for relieving nausea. It is commonly used to help women with morning sickness.

LIVER MERIDIAN

See page 50 for a full description of the Liver Meridian. The following point is commonly used in acupressure.

LV-3 *Tai Chong* (Great Rushing)

This point is located on top of the foot 1 cun below the web between the big toe and the second toe. It is a very important point, used for reducing tension and relaxing the body, and as a pathway to increase the flow of *qi*. It is generally used for clearing Liver stagnation, especially when someone is dealing with stress or feelings of frustration. At such a time you want to release the *qi*. When it is stimulated, this point helps regulate the flow of *qi*, relieving tension. It also helps to tonify Blood and *yin*.

Caution: IF YOU ARE PREGNANT, USE ONLY UNDER SUPERVISION FROM A TCM PRACTITIONER.

TRIPLE BURNER MERIDIAN

See page 48 for a full description of the Triple Burner Meridian. The following point is commonly used in acupressure.

TB-17 *Yi Feng* (Wind Screen)

Also known as SJ-17 (*San Jiao* 17), this point is located behind the earlobe. It is very good for reducing tinnitus (noise in the ears).

GALL BLADDER MERIDIAN

See page 49 for a full description of the Gall Bladder Meridian. The following points are those commonly used in acupressure.

GB-20 *Feng Chi* (Wind Pool)

This point is located on the neck muscle, midway between the base of the skull at the back of the head and the back of the ear. It is used for relaxation, and is especially useful for treating headaches, dizziness or a fuzzy head.

ACUPRESSURE CHART

⚠ Although useful for fertility treatment, these points should only be used during pregnancy under the supervision of a qualified TCM practitioner.

POINT	ABBREVIATION	WESTERN NAME	WARNING	NOTES
Conception Vessel (Ren mai)				
Zhong Ji	CV-3	Middle Pole		Used for acupuncture (pages 54–55)
Guan Yuan	CV-4	Gateway to Original Qi		
Qi Hai	CV-6	Sea of Qi		
Governing Vessel (Du mai)				
Yao Yang Guan	GV-3	Barrier of the Yang		
Large Intestine Meridian				
He Gu	LI-4	Joining Valley	⚠	
Qu Chi	LI-11	Pool at the Bend		Used for acupuncture (pages 54–55)
Stomach Meridian				
Tian Shu	ST-25	Heaven's Pivot		
Shui Dao	ST-28	Waterway	⚠	
Gui Lai	ST-29	Return	⚠	
Zu San Li	ST-36	Leg Three Miles		
Feng Long	ST-40	Abundant Bulge		Used for acupuncture (pages 54–55)
Jie Xi	ST-41	Stream Divide		Used for acupuncture (pages 54–55)
Spleen Meridian				
San Yin Jiao	SP-6	Three Yin Intersection	⚠	
Yin Ling Quan	SP-9	Yin Mound Spring		
Xue Hai	SP-10	Sea of Blood	⚠	
Urinary Bladder Meridian				
Ge Shu	UB-17	Diaphragm Shu		Used for acupuncture (pages 54–55)
Gan Shu	UB-18	Liver Shu		
Pi Shu	UB-20	Spleen Shu		
Shen Shu	UB-23	Kidney Shu		
Dachang Shu	UB-25	Large Intestine Shu		
Shang Liao	UB-31	Upper Crevice	⚠	
Ci Liao	UB-32	Second Crevice	⚠	
Zhong Liao	UB-33	Middle Crevice	⚠	
Xia Liao	UB-34	Lower Crevice	⚠	
Zhi Yin	UB-67	Reaching Yin	⚠	See description of point on page 234
Kidney Meridian				
Tai Xi	KID-3	Supreme Stream		Used for acupuncture (pages 54–55)
Zhao Hai	KID-6	Shining Sea		Used for acupuncture (pages 54–55)
Da He	KID-12	Great Luminance		Used for acupuncture (pages 54–55)
Pericardium Meridian				
Nei Guan	PC-6	Inner Pass		
Triple Burner Meridian (San Jiao)				
Yi Feng	TB-17	Wind Screen		
Gall Bladder Meridian				
Feng Chi	GB-20	Wind Pool		
Jian Jing	GB-21	Shoulder Well	⚠	
Liver Meridian				
Tai Chong	LV-3	Great Rushing	⚠	
Extra points				
Yin Tang	EX-HN 3	Hall of Impression		See illustration of point on page 232
Tai Yang	EX-HN 5	Great Sun		See illustration of point on page 232

USEFUL ACUPRESSURE POINTS FOR TCM HOME TREATMENT

	CONSTIPATION	INCONTINENCE URINARY DISORDERS	PAINFUL PERIODS	IRREGULAR PERIODS AMENORRHEA	RELAXATION HEADACHES	MORNING SICKNESS	IMPOTENCE	INSOMNIA ANXIETY	FATIGUE	TINNITUS	STRESS REDUCTION	DIGESTIVE PROBLEMS	BACKACHE
				✓									
		✓		✓			✓		✓				
			✓	✓			✓		✓				
		✓	✓	✓			✓						✓
			✓		✓								
	✓		✓									✓	
			✓										
			✓	✓			✓						
	✓		✓						✓			✓	
			✓	✓				✓					
		✓	✓										
			✓	✓									
					✓						✓		
												✓	
		✓							✓				✓
	✓								✓				✓
				✓									✓
				✓									✓
				✓									✓
				✓									✓
						✓							
										✓			
					✓								
					✓								
					✓				✓		✓		
					✓			✓					
			✓		✓								

GB-21 *Jian Jing* (Shoulder Well)

This point is located halfway between the tip of the shoulder and the base of the neck, at the highest point. It is used to aid relaxation, and to release muscle and neck ache.

Caution: IF YOU ARE PREGNANT, USE ONLY UNDER SUPERVISION FROM A TCM PRACTITIONER.

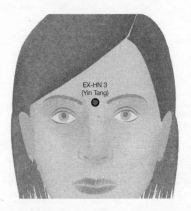

EX-HN 3
(Yin Tang)

EXTRAORDINARY HEAD-NECK POINTS

There are as many as 48 extraordinary 'extra' acupuncture points that are not included within the main meridians. They are not connected to one another – so it would be hard to illustrate them all. There are two 'extra' points that I find very useful and therefore recommend for home use with acupressure. The following points can be very helpful to promote relaxation.

EX-HN 3 *Yin Tang* (Hall of Impression)

This point is found midway between the inner edges of the eyebrows. It is used to treat insomnia and headaches, is good for treating dizziness and has a calming effect. The point can be pressed or stroked firmly for several minutes.

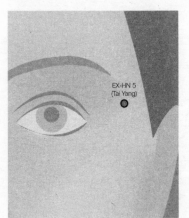

EX-HN 5
(Tai Yang)

EX-HN 5 *Tai Yang* (Great Sun)

This point is easily located near the temples, in the indentation that occurs near the outside of the eyebrow. This is the point that we naturally tend to soothe when suffering from tension. Applying pressure here is good for relaxation, particularly if you suffer from PMS and headaches.

Moxibustion

One of the key elements of TCM is the use of moxibustion. Moxa is another name for mugwort (*Artemisia vulgaris*), a common herb that is renowned for its healing properties. It has been used for centuries in China as an integral

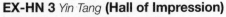

part of TCM, especially with acupuncture. These days it is used mainly in the form of candles. It is a very warming and very powerful herb used in the treatment of *yang* deficiency. When used properly, moxa can have an immediate effect.

Moxibustion is often used to help expel Cold from the body or tonify a deficiency of the Spleen, Stomach or Kidney so it is a useful tool for regulating the female menstrual cycle, warming a Cold uterus and soothing menstrual cramps. In men it can sometimes be appropriate to use it to promote sperm production, depending on individual diagnosis.

I don't use moxa as often as some practitioners; only when I am completely certain that it will make a difference.

USE MOXIBUSTION WITH CARE

Chinese medicine is quite sophisticated and different practitioners have different levels of skill. It is very important to consult someone who is properly qualified in the use of moxibustion as there are mild side effects if it is not used properly that may cause *yin* and *yang* imbalance.

If you suffer any of the following symptoms, you need to be cautious and consult a qualified practitioner: interrupted sleep, frequent thirst, a red tongue with a lack of coating, excess sweating or a short menstrual cycle if you are a woman.

WHAT TO EXPECT

Moxa is supplied as a large stick looking rather like a big cigar. It is used either on its own or in conjunction with acupuncture. The smoke from a moxa candle is healthy, but I must admit the smell is very unpleasant. For that reason we rarely use it in my clinic.

Nowadays, some companies make small moxa sticks; some of them are smokeless and can be used in clinics without too much disruption. I often use smokeless moxa with acupuncture, as it can be put on the tip of an acupuncture needle. I also show patients how to use moxibustion safely, so they can do it on their own at home – but only when it is necessary and appropriate.

HOW TO USE MOXIBUSTION AT HOME

Only use genuine moxa candles, as supplied by your TCM practitioner. Use it only on acupressure points shown to you by your TCM practitioner and use it for no more than 15 minutes a day.

1. Light the moxa herbal candle.

2. Release the smoke into the moxa jar, until there is no air in the jar.

3. Introduce the heated jar to the acupressure point on the body (without touching) and then move it away. The idea is to warm rather than burn the body with the heat.

4. Gently warm, then take away, warm, then take away.

5. Continue in the same way for about 15 minutes.

Caution: MOXIBUSTION SHOULD ONLY BE USED UNDER THE CAREFUL GUIDANCE OF A QUALIFIED PRACTITIONER.

I do not recommend that patients use the 'cupping' technique that some practitioners use. This is unnecessary and can be unsafe in untutored hands.

USING MOXIBUSTION TO TURN A BREECH BABY

I most commonly use moxibustion in the case of a baby who is lying in the breech position prior to birth, as the heat of the moxa candle used on particular acupuncture points can encourage the baby to turn. This is the time when I guide patients to use moxa at home as it must be done every day until the baby has turned.

A baby is said to be in the breech position when he or she is head-up instead of head-down in the womb, which can cause problems at birth. About 18 per cent of babies lie this way until week 37 of pregnancy. Most breech babies will turn spontaneously before or during labour without any assistance, but about 3 to 4 per cent may need help to turn. TCM practitioners will often use moxa to help turn the baby, with great success. A clinical trial is currently underway which is expected to verify the efficacy of this method.

The acupuncture point used is on the Urinary Bladder Meridian. It is UB-67 *Zhi Yin* (Reaching *Yin*), located on the outside of the end of the small toe, just outside the corner of the nail. This is an important point because it is where the Urinary Bladder Meridian and the Kidney Meridian connect. This point is therefore able to regulate the Kidney and tonify *qi*.

Many acupuncturists show pregnant mothers how to use moxa on this point, very gently, for 15 minutes a day to encourage the baby to turn into the correct position for birth.

Chapter 11

BEING PREGNANT

Pregnancy brings many wonderful joys and excitement. However, many women are surprised to discover that the hormonal adjustments cause them to experience a variety of symptoms and discomfort.

For example, many women report at least one food craving during pregnancy for sweet, salty, spicy or sour foods; some even crave non-food substances such as laundry starch (a condition called pica). Many of these cravings seem to come from nowhere and are overpowering. No one knows for sure what causes them (some women going through the menopause experience similar strong food cravings and aversions). It is possible that extreme hormonal changes during pregnancy have an impact on taste and smell; however, it may also be a signal that there is a deficiency of one nutrient or another that needs to be replenished. There is an old saying that a pregnant woman who craves spicy foods will have a girl; and a woman who craves sour foods will have a boy – but of course, there is no proof in the statement. To date, there is no scientific evidence for a link between cravings and nutritional requirements either.

The first trimester (weeks 1–13)

The first trimester is the most critical time in a pregnancy because the early stages of foetal development often influence whether the pregnancy will go full term.

Your baby will grow and develop very quickly in the first trimester. By the 10th week of pregnancy all the body parts are present (although they are not quite fully developed) and the placenta is fully formed. At this point, the embryo is known as a foetus. Nutrients are transferred from you to the baby through the placenta and waste products from the baby are removed via your blood circulation.

By the 12th week, your baby will be about 6 cm (2½ inches) long. At this stage the eyelids are still sealed shut and the ears are forming but your baby's forehead is growing to accommodate the developing brain.

Some women may not feel any different; missed periods may be the only outward sign that something out of the ordinary is going on. But hormones are causing other changes to a woman's body too. One early symptom is breast tenderness. You may also notice an increased need to pass urine because your growing womb starts to press on your bladder, and the hormonal changes may make you feel very tired. Many women feel sick in the early stages of pregnancy; some worse in the morning, but it can happen any time or throughout the day.

SUMMARY OF THE FIRST TRIMESTER

For most women, the first trimester is a time of discomfort, due to the many physical and hormonal changes that occur, with many suffering from:

- Morning sickness
- Fatigue
- Breast enlargement
- More frequent urination
- Constipation

For more information about these conditions, see pages 242–243.

Folic acid

The current health authority guidelines suggest that a pregnant woman should take folic acid supplements (see pages 196–197) at least every day for the first 12 weeks of pregnancy, but I would say there is no harm in taking it until the baby is born. The first trimester is the time when the baby's brain and nervous system develop. Folic acid (see page 193) reduces the chance of the baby being born with a spinal cord problem called a neural tube defect (NTD). If you believe you are at a high risk of having a baby with a NTD, you should take professional advice.

LOOK AFTER YOUR BODY

- Avoid drinking alcohol during pregnancy. This is particularly important during the first three months, when the baby's most important organs are forming.
- Slow down a bit if you exercise regularly, particularly if you have miscarried before.
- Do not carry anything heavy that overuses your abdominal muscles.
- Get as much sleep and relaxation as you can.

All-important rest

The first three months of pregnancy are associated with a time of great change inside the body and this process should not be strained or aggravated by increased or excessive movement. It is not surprising that a pregnant woman feels tired or fatigued during the first trimester and my recommendation is to try to rest as much as you can during this time. I do, however, encourage pregnant women to feel free to express themselves creatively because it is an empowering and uniquely expressive time that marks new beginnings.

The primary task of the woman during the first three months is to remain calm and in good health. It is important to get enough sleep in a peaceful environment.

TCM AND THE FIRST TRIMESTER

Nausea and vomiting are the result of the growing foetus stimulating the circulation of *qi* in the uterus. Stomach *qi*, which usually descends, will instead rebel upwards causing nausea and vomiting. The nausea may be triggered by an aversion to a food smell or by an intake of food and is often accompanied by weariness and shortness of breath.

Where there is a simultaneous stagnation of Liver *qi* these troubles can be exaggerated because the Liver governs *qi* flow via the blood and sinew to the embryo during this phase of pregnancy.

Women who have pre-existing liver *qi* stagnation may in addition suffer from mood swings and a bitter taste in the mouth, as a result of a disharmony between the Liver and Stomach, causing both Liver and Stomach *qi* to rebel upwards instead of downwards.

In some women, Stomach *qi* may rebel upwards together with retained Phlegm as a result of a predisposed Spleen deficiency. These women typically vomit sputum and saliva, experience a suffocating feeling in the chest and a tasteless sensation in the mouth.

I often prescribe *Xiang Sha Lui Jun Tang* formula at this time, which promotes *qi* throughout the body and ensures the Blood flow supports the developing pregnancy. The formula strengthens the digestive function, reduces Phlegm, Damp and morning sickness. My aim is to support the mother so that she can provide the Blood and Kidney essence that are required to nourish the foetus. In addition, it is important to keep the lower abdomen in good form with good blood circulation.

Not all pregnant women will experience morning sickness or vomiting, and not all will experience frequent urination, like most pregnancy books suggest. Most of our patients just carry on as normal and hardly slow down at all. Our female patients often find that by using TCM treatments or preparations, they produce healthier eggs and have more peaceful pregnancies. I would like to think that the babies are healthier too.

The second trimester (weeks 14–26)

This trimester is sometimes called the 'honeymoon period' because during the second trimester a woman usually starts to feel better. Typically, morning sickness tapers off or stops completely and emotions become less erratic. However, some women experience a number of minor ailments which can cause varying degrees of discomfort.

Your breasts will continue to enlarge and you might feel lightheaded or dizzy at times. Your baby will become more active now and undergo rapid growth, causing the surrounding ligaments to stretch; as a result you will start to experience abdominal aches. Your pregnancy will start to show and as your shape changes you may worry about the long-term effects that pregnancy will have on your body.

SUMMARY OF THE SECOND TRIMESTER

For many women, this is an easier trimester, though some symptoms of pregnancy will persist and others become apparent:

- Continued breast enlargement
- Yellow liquid (colostrum) may leak from the nipples
- Quickening or initial movement of baby felt by the mother
- Increased abdominal size due to enlarging uterus
- Constipation
- Emotional vulnerability
- Breathlessness
- Varicose veins
- Dizziness
- Heartburn

For more information about these conditions, see pages 244–247.

Your baby's progress

By week 16, all your baby's body parts have fully formed and there is a strong heartbeat. The ears are functioning and your developing baby is sleeping and swallowing. You might start to feel your baby kick as he or she becomes more active. This is also a time of rapid growth.

During this time you will be given an ultrasound scan to gather valuable information about the progress of your pregnancy and your baby's health, which includes an assessment of your baby's location. (Do not panic if your baby lies in a breech or transverse position. Many babies lie this way and correct themselves by the time of delivery.)

At 18 weeks your baby's blood vessels are visible through the thin skin, and the ears are now in their final position, although they will still stand out from the head a bit. Unseen by the naked eye, a protective covering of myelin is beginning to form around the nerves, which increases the speed at which they send messages to and from the brain; this process will continue for a year after your baby is born.

If you are having a girl, her uterus and fallopian tubes are formed now and in place. If you are having a boy, his genitals will be noticeable now, though they may be hidden during an ultrasound.

TCM AND THE SECOND TRIMESTER

During this trimester the formation of your baby's stomach and intestines are completed. In addition, you can see the changes in your body and feel the movement of your child. During this phase your Blood and *qi* must be strengthened more and more so a good diet and regular mealtimes are important, as well as having enough sleep, regular exercise and avoiding getting cold. Pregnancy-related vomiting during this time signals a tendency towards stagnation. Harmony is important now. Most women experience this time as pleasant and powerful.

In the majority of cases (approximately 95 per cent), herbal medication can be suspended at this point and the pregnancy should be secure. I keep very few patients on herbal medication during this trimester; only those who have experienced repeated miscarriage in the past. On one occasion I treated a woman who had miscarried repeatedly; one pregnancy ended at five months. When she conceived again, she had slight blood spotting. I therefore resumed herbal treatment until the bleeding stopped during the seventh month of pregnancy.

Acupuncture treatment is still recommended for most women to ensure that they and their baby are in good form to sail through the rest of their 40-week journey. The sessions do not, however, need to be as regular and intensive as before you became pregnant. My recommendation during the second trimester is to have acupuncture every two or three weeks, depending on how well you feel and how much help you feel you need.

The third trimester (weeks 27–40)

During the last trimester of pregnancy, there might be very contrasting experiences. You are on the homeward stretch and although some women still feel the 'bloom' of pregnancy, many feel very tired and uncomfortable. Not only are you carrying a lot of extra weight as your baby is growing more and more, your expanding uterus also rearranges other organs in your body, adding extra strain. You might also feel thirsty, but still need to go to the bathroom often.

SUMMARY OF THE THIRD TRIMESTER

Typical characteristics of the third trimester include:

- Lower back pain
- Continued movements of the baby that can be seen and felt in the belly
- The abdomen becomes firm to the touch
- Swelling of extremities (feet, ankles and fingers)
- Continued fatigue
- Sleeping problems
- Painless contractions (Braxton Hicks)

For more information about these conditions, see pages 247–250.

Your baby's progress

By week 27, your baby will weigh around 1.1 kg (2¼ lb) and measure about 37 cm (14½ inches) from the top of the head to the heels. Your baby can now blink his or her eyes, which will have eyelashes. With their eyesight developing, light that filters in through your womb might be visible. Billions of neurons are developing in the brain and your baby will be adding more body fat in preparation for life in the outside world.

Your baby's muscles and lungs are continuing to mature, and the head is growing bigger to make room for the developing brain.

By week 31 your baby is heading into a growth spurt. He or she will be able to turn the head from side to side, and the arms, legs and body are beginning to plump out as necessary fat accumulates underneath the skin. As your baby is becoming more active, you may have trouble sleeping because the kicking and somersaulting will keep you awake. However, all this moving is a sign that your baby is active and healthy.

The bones of your baby's skull are not yet fused, which allows them to overlap if your birth canal is a snug fit during labour.

This is the reason that your baby may have a cone-shaped head after birth, but the effect is normal and temporary. It is called 'moulding'.

WHAT YOUR BABY NEEDS FROM YOU

To meet your baby's increasing nutritional demands, you will need to eat plenty of protein, vitamin C, folic acid and iron, as well as calcium because your baby's bones will be soaking up a lot of calcium as the skeleton is hardening.

Early births

If you have been nervous about premature labour you will be relieved to know that babies born between 34 and 37 weeks with no other health problems are generally fine. They may have a few short-term health issues, but in the long run they usually do just as well as full-term babies.

If you go into labour during week 37 your baby's lungs are likely to be mature enough to function fully outside the womb. Some babies need a little more time – if you are planning to have a repeat caesarean-section, this would be scheduled between 37 and 39 weeks unless there is a medical reason to intervene earlier.

From week 37 to week 40 your baby will be considered full-term; after week 40 it will be considered post-term.

TCM AND THE THIRD TRIMESTER

From the Chinese medicine viewpoint, the third trimester is the preparation time for the separation of mother and child. During this time advice generally focuses on encouraging movement to promote the circulation of *qi* and Blood by means of gentle exercise such as walking. Although regular movement is considered strengthening, caution is advised for women who had difficulty getting pregnant: they should not engage in too much dynamic activity to avoid endangering the holding and nourishing of the child. Nevertheless, all women, especially those who had difficulty getting pregnant, are reassured by the thought that they have managed to reach this stage.

During this time anything that nourishes the Kidney is regarded as beneficial, such as plenty of sleep, good nutritious food and warmth, particularly warm feet, knees and back. These recommendations are especially important for women who had difficulty conceiving due to a constitutional Kidney deficiency, because it is gathering *jing* that is extremely important to make your child healthy.

Acupuncture

Acupuncture can be a very effective and safe treatment option during the third trimester of pregnancy. It is particularly effective in treating sleeplessness, back pain, sciatica, high blood pressure and swelling.

Qi and Blood stagnation are the most common causes of backache in pregnancy. In this case the backache is typically acute and the pain severe, stabbing, worse with rest and better with movement.

During pregnancy and childbirth, a lot of extra strain is placed on the back, both from extra weight and consumption of Kidney *qi*, especially in women with a constitutional weakness. Therefore, backache can also be the result of consumption of Kidney essence, manifesting typically as a chronic ache that is better with rest and worse with exertion.

Extreme climatic factors such as cold and damp can also cause backache as these easily invade, especially the Urinary Bladder Meridian, causing blockage of the meridian and obstruction of the flow of *qi* and Blood. Therefore great care should be taken to wear adequate clothing. Here the ache is typically aggravated by cold and relieved by warmth.

Pregnancy symptoms and treatments

These are some of the symptoms you may experience during pregnancy, with some ideas for treatments.

MORNING SICKNESS

Many pregnant women experience some nausea and vomiting during the first trimester of pregnancy; this often eases off around the beginning of the second trimester. These symptoms are an unpleasant and often incapacitating side effect of pregnancy. The cause is unknown, but some research suggests it may be related to high levels of pregnancy hormones. There are things you can do to try and reduce the nausea and sickness: get plenty of rest, eat little and often, stay calm and relaxed, and avoid smells and tastes that make you feel queasy.

Morning sickness has been reported to have a positive effect on pregnancy outcome and is associated with a decreased risk of miscarriage. However, if you are suffering from severe, excessive or protracted vomiting, you are at risk of dehydration and need to seek medical advice. You should also see your doctor or midwife if you can't keep any food or fluid down.

Nausea can be eased by drinking apple juice, warm water with lemon or warm water with honey.

FATIGUE

Some women feel tired throughout pregnancy, whereas others hardly seem to slow down at all. Increased fatigue is particularly common during the first trimester and tends to return in late pregnancy. What causes it is uncertain, but it may be related to:

- Physiological and psychological changes occurring in the body. These include foetal growth and development; and hormonal changes, in particular a dramatic rise in progesterone.
- Morning sickness, which can be depleting.
- Increased frequency of urination. It can be hard to get a good night's sleep if you are getting up to use the bathroom more frequently.
- Anxiety.
- Other health problems, such as an underactive thyroid or anaemia.

Here are some simple steps you might like to try to beat the fatigue:

Get plenty of rest Start by going to bed a little earlier than usual and if possible, take a short nap during the day. Putting your head down for 10 to 15 minutes can do wonders.

Eat healthily A healthy diet made up of vegetables, fruit, fish and chicken can be energizing, while providing you with all the nutrition you need. Do not forget you need about 300 extra calories every day now.

Remain hydrated Drink plenty of water during the day. If frequent urination wakes you up at night, drink plenty during the day but cut back a few hours before you go to bed.

Breathe deeply This will increase your oxygen intake.

Keep moving Take moderate exercise, such as a short walk, every day – unless advised otherwise. Stretching frequently throughout the day can also help.

Be patient If you are at the beginning of your pregnancy, you will soon be in your second trimester by which time most women feel better again.

If you still feel tired, ask your doctor for a routine blood test to check for other potential health problems.

INCREASED URINATION

The need to urinate more frequently is one of the most common early signs of pregnancy, starting in about week 6. Hormonal changes cause an increased blood flow through your kidneys, which results in your bladder filling more often. Moreover, over the course of your pregnancy, the amount of blood in your body rises by about

50 per cent, which obviously leads to a lot of extra fluid being processed by your kidneys and ending up in your bladder.

As your uterus grows it puts pressure on your bladder, which further compounds the problem. Going to the bathroom may not always offer relief from the feeling of urgency. However, do not go thirsty in an attempt to reduce your bathroom visits, instead avoid beverages that have a mild diuretic effect, such as coffee and tea, which you should be drinking in very limited amounts anyway. Drinking plenty of fluids during the day and cutting back in the hours before going to bed might be worth a try, though it might not bring you relief.

BREAST ENLARGEMENT

Breast growth and other tissue changes are a result of hormone levels rising, in preparation for lactation. Your breasts may continue to grow throughout pregnancy and your bra size may go up a cup size or two, especially if it is your first baby.

CONSTIPATION

Constipation is a common problem during pregnancy and as many as half of pregnant women suffer from it at some point. One cause is an increase in the hormone progesterone, which relaxes smooth muscles throughout the body, including those in the digestive tract. As a result, food passes through the intestines more slowly. Later in pregnancy the pressure exerted by the growing uterus on the rectum may further exaggerate the problem. Constipation can be worsened by taking iron supplements, particularly in high doses.

A woman can suffer from constipation during any of the three trimesters. From the Chinese medicine viewpoint, constipation may be due to a number of factors. During the first trimester constipation is often a result of stagnant *qi* or Heat in the intestines, while during the second trimester it is usually due to a deficiency of Blood leading to insufficient fluids to moisten the stool.

- Constipation due to Heat: the stool is dry, accompanied by restlessness and a dry mouth. This is a result of the Heat consuming body fluids hence drying the stool, while the upward rising of Heat may cause a dry mouth and restlessness.
- Constipation due to *qi* stagnation: this is frequently accompanied by belching but the stool is not dry.
- Constipation due to excessive Cold and *qi* stagnation: this indicates a deficiency of *yang qi*. A deficiency of Blood leads to malnourishment, causing difficult bowel movements and resulting in a dull complexion. During pregnancy especially, Kidney *qi* is required by the growing foetus. Women with a *qi* deficiency commonly complain of breathlessness or shortness of breath.

244

TIPS TO PREVENT OR EASE CONSTIPATION

- Try to eat high-fibre foods every day, such as wholegrain foods, fresh fruit and vegetables.
- Drink plenty of water – at least six to eight glasses a day. Some people find that drinking warm water first thing in the morning helps to get things moving. Fruit juice, especially prune juice, can also be helpful.
- Regular exercise such as walking or swimming can ease constipation and leave you feeling more fit and healthy.
- Your bowels are most likely to be active after a meal, especially in the morning. Make time to use the bathroom and never put it off when you feel the urge.
- If you are taking a multi-vitamin that contains a large dose of iron and you are not anaemic, talk to your healthcare provider about switching to a supplement with less iron.
- Acupuncture can be a tremendous help in getting your bowels moving.

VARICOSE VEINS

Varicose veins appear as enlarged blue or purple veins that may bulge near the surface of the skin and are most likely to show up in your legs. They are a result of your growing uterus putting pressure on the large vein on the right side of your body (called the inferior vena cava). This increases the pressure in the other veins of your leg, which are already working hard, and against gravity, because they return blood to your heart from your feet.

In addition, when you are pregnant the amount of blood in your body increases and your progesterone levels rise; this causes the walls of your blood vessels to relax, which adds to the burden on your veins. They may give you little or no discomfort, or they may make your legs ache or feel heavy and the skin around them may itch, throb or feel like it is burning. The symptoms tend to be worse at the end of the day, especially if you have been on your feet for hours. Try to rest often, preferably with your feet in an elevated position.

DIZZINESS

It is common to feel lightheaded or dizzy when you are pregnant. This is because your cardiovascular system undergoes dramatic changes. Your heart rate increases, your heart pumps more blood per minute and the amount of blood in your veins almost doubles.

During a normal pregnancy, your blood pressure gradually decreases, reaching its lowest point in the middle part of your pregnancy. After that it begins to rise, returning to its regular level by the end of pregnancy. Most of the time, the cardiovascular and nervous systems are able to adjust to these natural changes. However, occasionally they do not, which can leave you feeling lightheaded or a bit dizzy. If you actually faint, it could be a sign that something is wrong and you must seek medical advice.

Here are a few tips to help you cope:

- If you feel dizzy, try to lie down as soon as possible so that you do not fall and hurt yourself.
- You can prevent lightheadedness during pregnancy by lying on your side instead of flat on your back so that your uterus does not further compress the vena cava.
- Avoid standing up too fast and thus causing your blood pressure to drop.
- Try not to get dehydrated and ensure you eat enough or eat small, frequent meals during the day to prevent your blood sugar level from getting too low.
- Although keeping fit is good, excessive exercise should be avoided as it can make you feel faint or lower your blood pressure too much. This caution also applies to having a hot shower or bath.

BREATHLESSNESS

Becoming breathless even when doing mundane activities like walking to the bathroom is perfectly normal now. Your growing uterus is crowding your lungs, making it harder for air to flow in and out. So try to slow down and take it easy. However, if you find that your shortness of breath is becoming severe, please consult your doctor.

EMOTIONAL VULNERABILITY

Although pregnancy is often portrayed as a time of great joy, you will probably also start worrying or feel fearful about what you eat, drink, think, feel and do, because you don't want to do anything that could hurt your developing baby. You may also worry about how your baby will change your life and personal relationships. This is perfectly normal and natural.

Avoid carrying your anxiety alone; share your fears with your partner, friends or family members. Other parents-to-be will also be a source of support because they are probably experiencing the same anxieties. However, if you have a specific reason to be concerned about your baby's health then share your concerns with your doctor or midwife.

HEARTBURN

Many women experience heartburn and other gastrointestinal discomforts, especially during the second half of pregnancy. Although this is common and generally harmless, it can be quite uncomfortable. Heartburn, also called acid reflux, is a burning sensation which often extends from the bottom of the breastbone to the lower throat. This is caused by some of the hormonal and physical changes that take place in your body during pregnancy. For example, the hormone progesterone relaxes the valve that separates the oesophagus from the stomach, allowing gastric acids to seep back up and cause that unpleasant burning sensation.

Later in pregnancy your growing baby crowds your abdominal cavity, pushing further stomach acids back into the oesophagus. So unfortunately, heartburn will usually come and go until your baby is born. However, you can take steps to minimize it:

- Avoid fatty, spicy and citrus foods that cause you digestive distress, such as chocolate, citrus fruits and juices, tomatoes, mustard, vinegar, processed meat and pâtés, fried foods, curries and chilli.
- Avoid alcohol, especially strong beer, sparkling wine and white wine.
- Avoid eating big meals. Instead, eat several small meals throughout the day.
- Take your time when eating and chew thoroughly.
- Drink plenty of water throughout the day, but avoid drinking large quantities during meals because this can distend your stomach.
- Avoid eating late at night, or close to bedtime; instead allow two to three hours for digestion before lying down.
- You might find it more comfortable in bed to elevate your upper body with several pillows, which will help to keep your stomach acids where they belong and will aid your digestion.

LOWER BACK PAIN

Most pregnant women experience back pain at some point during their pregnancy, but it appears most often during the third trimester (or becomes worse as pregnancy progresses). A combination of your growing uterus and hormonal changes are usually to blame for your aching back. Your growing uterus shifts your centre of gravity, as well as stretching and weakening your abdominal muscles; this changes your posture and puts strain on your back. Your pain may even increase if there is additional pressure on a nerve.

You are also carrying extra weight, which puts increased pressure on your joints and makes the muscles work harder, which is why your back may feel worse at the end of the day.

The hormonal changes in pregnancy loosen the joints and the ligaments that attach the pelvic bones to the spine. This can make you feel less stable and cause pain when you walk, stand or sit for long periods, or when you lift things.

Your back may continue to hurt for a few months after giving birth, but once your muscles regain their strength and your joints become less lax, it will dissipate. A long or difficult labour may also cause you to end up with a sore back. You can help recovery by being conscious of a good posture, and always bending from your knees when lifting objects and children to minimize the stress on your back. If at all possible, try also to get some help with childcare to prevent the exhaustion and stress you may experience taking care of a newborn baby 24 hours a day. Stress can make it harder to recover from aches and pains after childbirth.

SWELLING OF EXTREMITIES

A certain amount of swelling in the ankles and feet during pregnancy is normal; it is sometimes accompanied by mild swelling of the hands. This is caused by water retention and by changes in blood chemistry that cause some fluid to be relocated in tissue. In addition, the growing uterus puts pressure on the pelvic veins and vena cava, which carries blood from the lower limbs back to the heart. This pressure slows down the return flow of blood from the legs, causing it to pool and forcing fluid from the veins into the tissues of the feet and ankles.

Here are a few tips to minimize the swelling:

- Since the vena cava is on the right side of the body, you can help relieve the increased pressure on your veins by lying on your left side.
- Put your feet up whenever possible and do not cross your legs or ankles while sitting.
- Stretch your legs frequently while sitting; rotate your ankles and wiggle your toes.
- Wear comfortable shoes that stretch to accommodate swelling and do not wear socks or stockings that have tight bands around the ankles. Waist-high maternity support stockings may be a further option to prevent blood from pooling around the ankles.
- Drinking plenty of water actually helps your body retain less water.
- Take regular exercise such as walking or swimming and avoid sitting or standing too long, to help keep the blood circulating.
- Most of all, try not to let the swelling get you down. Once you have given birth, the swelling will disappear fairly rapidly as your body eliminates the excess fluid.

Oedema (swelling) during the third trimester is common and is often worse during the summer. However, if you notice swelling in your face, puffiness around your eyes, more than slight swelling of your hands or excessive or sudden swelling of your feet or ankles then you should call your midwife or doctor because this could be a sign of pre-eclampsia, a serious condition.

PRE-ECLAMPSIA

Pre-eclampsia causes the blood vessels to constrict, resulting in high blood pressure and reduced blood flow, which can affect the vital organs, such as the liver, kidneys and brain; it can also affect the uterus, which can mean problems for your baby. The changes in the blood vessels may cause capillaries to 'leak' fluid into the tissues causing swelling, while tiny blood vessels in the kidneys leak protein in the urine.

Pre-eclampsia most commonly appears at 37 weeks, but it can develop any time in the second half of pregnancy, including during labour or even after delivery. It can range from mild to severe and progress slowly or rapidly. The only way to recover from pre-eclampsia is to deliver your baby.

TROUBLE SLEEPING

You are bound to have trouble sleeping at some point during your pregnancy, particularly during the first or last trimesters. During the first trimester it might be nausea or a constant need to go to the bathroom that may keep you from a good night's sleep. Later in pregnancy you may suffer from heartburn or breathlessness and find it more comfortable to sleep with your upper body propped up. During your third trimester you may find it helpful to sleep on your side with your legs bent and a pillow between your knees; place one more pillow under your belly and another behind your back. Regular exercise makes you healthier both physically and mentally, and can improve sleep too.

PAINLESS CONTRACTIONS (BRAXTON HICKS)

Braxton Hicks contractions are sporadic uterine contractions that start during the first trimester, though they are not usually felt until sometime after mid-pregnancy, if at all. They were first described in 1872 by John Braxton Hicks, an English doctor, hence their name.

Braxton Hicks contractions usually remain infrequent, irregular and painless, until the last few weeks of pregnancy when they tend to occur more often and are hard to distinguish from the real thing. Braxton Hicks contractions may be intermittently rhythmic, relatively close together, and even painful. However, unlike true labour, the contractions don't grow consistently longer, stronger and closer together.

If you have not reached 37 weeks yet and your contractions are becoming more frequent, rhythmic or painful, or if you have any of these possible signs of preterm labour, you should call your doctor immediately:

- Menstrual-like cramping or more than four contractions in an hour.
- More than usual vaginal discharge, or a change in the type of discharge.
- Vaginal bleeding or spotting.
- Increased pelvic pressure.
- Dull or rhythmic lower backache, especially if it is a new problem for you.

If you have passed 37 weeks there is usually no need to call your doctor just for contractions until they last about 60 seconds each and are five minutes apart, unless of course you have been advised differently by your doctor.

DEALING WITH BRAXTON HICKS

To make Braxton Hicks contractions less uncomfortable when you are within a few weeks of your due date, you might like to try these measures:

- Sometimes walking helps, while at other times resting eases contractions, so try changing your activity or position to bring relief. In contrast, true labour contractions will persist and progress regardless of what you do.
- A warm bath (not too hot) may help your body relax and ease Braxton Hicks contractions.
- Braxton Hicks contractions can sometimes be brought on by dehydration, so drinking a couple of glasses of water may help.
- Slow, deep breathing may help you cope with the discomfort of the Braxton Hicks contractions.

Appendix

WHAT TO EXPECT WHEN YOU VISIT YOUR FERTILITY DOCTOR

The initial consultation is a chance for your doctor to get to know you. It is very helpful if you prepare all the relevant information before the visit so your doctor has all he or she needs to advise you on what help can be offered to you, what your options are and what tests or investigations may be needed before your treatment plan is finalized.

I know it is hard as many patients find it difficult to bring up this painful subject. However, you are looking for a helping hand and it is important not to waste this most important consultation, which could be crucial for you. I have prepared below a checklist of questions which your doctor or fertility clinic will probably ask. This is an example of the questionnaire we ask our new patients to fill out at my clinic.

PATIENT REGISTRATION

Female		**Male**	
Surname		Surname	
First name		First name	
DOB	Age	DOB	Age
Height	Weight	Height	Weight
Occupation		Occupation	

(You must fill in both partners' details)
Your home address and contact details
Your family doctor's name and address
Your hospital or fertility clinic doctor's name and address
Consent for your family doctor to be informed of your treatment progress.

QUESTIONS FOR BOTH OF YOU

How long have you been together without contraception?

[In other words, how long have you been having unprotected intercourse? This is different from asking, 'How long have you been trying to conceive?' I do not like my patients to use the word 'trying' as it tends to lead to arguments between the couple about whether or not they have been trying hard enough. Common sense tells us that a natural conception should come naturally; so it is not because you are not trying that you cannot conceive but because there may be an underlying problem that causes a delay in conceiving or prevents the pregnancy occurring.]

QUESTIONS FOR THE WOMAN

Do you smoke?
If yes, how many cigarettes do you smoke per day?
If yes, how many years have you been smoking?
If no, have you ever smoked?
If yes, how many cigarettes did you smoke per day?
If yes, how many years did you smoke?

Do you drink alcohol?
If yes, how many units per week do you drink?

Do you have a special diet?
If yes, what diet are you on?
If yes, what reason are you on a special diet?
If yes, how long have you been on the special diet?
If yes, are you vegan or vegetarian?

General health
Have you had any allergies?
If yes, what are they?
Have you had any surgery in the past?
If yes, what and when?
Are you on any long-term medication?
If yes, give details.
Are you aware of any history of genetic/hereditary illness in your family?

Have you ever had any of the following (answer yes or no to each)?
HIV
Hepatitis B/C
Chlamydia
Asthma
Eczema
Migraine
High blood pressure

Herpes

Cystitis

Thyroid problems

Colitis

Epilepsy

Pelvic Inflammatory Disease (PID)

Abnormal smear tests

ME

Diabetes

Radiotherapy

Chemotherapy

If you have had any of the above, are they recurrent?

Previous obstetric history

Have you ever been pregnant?

If yes, was the pregnancy with your current partner?

If yes, how many pregnancies have you had? Please supply specific dates.

If yes, how many full-term pregnancies have you had?

If you have had a full-term pregnancy, how did you give birth? (Was the delivery by caesarean-section or vaginal?)

If you have had a full-term pregnancy, have you ever had any complications during or after the delivery?

Have you ever had a termination in the past?

If yes, when was it?

Have you experienced an ectopic pregnancy?

If yes, did you have your tube removed surgically?

Have you experienced a miscarriage?

If yes, how many miscarriages have you had?

If yes, at how many weeks did each miscarriage occur?

If yes, did you require an evacuation of retained products of conception (ERPC) after the miscarriage?

Have you had surgery to remove a fibroid?

Previous investigations

Have you had a laparoscopy and dye test?

Have you had a hysteroscopy?

Have you had a tubal patency test such as a hysterosalpingogram?

Have you had an ultrasound scan?

If yes, when was the latest scan you had?

Have you had any hormone tests?

Have you had Day 1–5 ovarian reserve test?

[This test includes FSH, LH, oestradiol and prolactin. Usually more than one test is performed as levels tend to fluctuate, particularly those of FSH and oestradiol.]

Have you had a Day 3 fertility potential test?
[This test includes Anti-Mullerian and Inhibin B hormone tests]
Have you had testosterone and thyroid function tests?
Have you had miscarriage screening, such as a blood clotting investigation?

Below is a form that will help you list all the tests you have had, in date order. It will be very helpful to your doctor to have all this information to hand when you visit, as it will allow more time for detailed discussion.

Test	Date:
Day 1–5 FSH	
Day 1–5 LH	
Day 1–5 oestradiol	
Day 1–5 prolactin	
Day 21 progesterone	
Day 3 Anti-Mullerian hormone	
Day 3 Inhibin B	
Testosterone	
TSH	
FT4	
FT3	
T4	
Thyroid Antibodies	

Your menstrual cycle
At what age did you start your periods?
How regular are they?
How regular have they been for the last two to three years?
How long is the shortest menstrual cycle?
How long is the longest menstrual cycle?
How many days does your period last?
Are your periods heavy, moderate or light in your own experience?
Do you notice clots in the menstrual discharge?
If yes, are there a lot of clots or just a few?
Do you suffer from period pain?
If yes, do you take painkillers?
Do you have inter-menstrual bleeding (between periods)?
If yes, how many days?
Do you have postmenstrual bleeding?
If yes, how many days?
Do you have post-coital bleeding?
If yes, how many days?
Do you have premenstrual bleeding?
If yes, how many days?
When was your last period (which date)?

QUESTIONS FOR THE MAN

Do you smoke?

If yes, how many cigarettes do you smoke per day?

If yes, how many years have you been smoking?

If no, have you ever smoked?

If yes, how many cigarettes did you smoke per day?

If yes, how many years did you smoke?

Do you drink alcohol?

If yes, how many units per week do you drink?

Do you have a special diet?

If yes, what diet are you on?

If yes, what reason are you on a special diet?

If yes, how long have you been on the special diet?

If yes, are you vegan or vegetarian?

Have you been the father of any pregnancy in the past?

If yes, did any go to full term? And do you have any children?

General health

Have you had any allergies?

If yes, what are they?

Have you had any surgery in the past?

If yes, what and when?

Are you on any long-term medication?

If yes, give details.

Have you had any illnesses or operations in the past?

Please indicate (with dates) any prescribed medication you have taken during the last 2 years (not including assisted fertility treatment).

Have you ever had any of the following (answer yes or no to each)?

HIV

Hepatitis B/C

Asthma

High blood pressure

Diabetes

Herpes

Thyroid problems

Colitis

Cystitis

Undescended testicle(s)

Surgery for hernia

Surgery for prostate problems

Testicular surgery

Testicular tumour
Varicocele
Mumps
Sexually transmitted disease
Vasectomy
Vasectomy reversal
Radiotherapy
Chemotherapy
Inflammation of the testicle or epididymis
If you have had any of the above, are they recurrent?

Sexual history
Do you have any sexual problems?
Are you able to produce a semen sample by masturbation?
Are you aware of any history of genetic/hereditary illness in your family?

Fertility investigation
Have you ever been diagnosed with a sperm problem?
Have you ever been advised to have a testicular biopsy?
Have you ever been advised to have a male hormone test?
Do you have a prostate problem?
Do you have erectile dysfunction?
Do you have an impotence problem?
Have you had any other surgery in the past?
If yes, what was it and when was the surgery carried out?

Semen analysis
If you have had any semen analysis, list the details below.
Date
Volume (ml)
Liquefaction
pH:
Count (in millions)
Motility (%)
Forward progression (%)
MAR IgA (%)
MAR IgG (%)
Round cells (in millions)
Abnormal form (%)
[For a couple who have had a long history of infertility, the following test results may be quite important.]
DNA fragmentation index (%)
High DNA sustainability (%)

PREVIOUS FERTILITY TREATMENTS

Female hormone treatment

Have you had Clomiphene ovulation induction in the past?

If yes, how many cycles have you had?

Have you had super-ovulation induction in the past?

If yes, how many cycles have you had?

Have you ever been prescribed Metformin?

If yes, how long have you been on it?

Male hormone treatment

Have you had any hormonal treatment?

If yes, what was it and for how long did you receive treatment?

Details of assisted fertility treatment

(include IUI, IVF and ICSI)

Date	Cycle	No: Follicles/eggs/embryos	Endometrium	Pregnancy

[In my clinic, I am particularly interested in the scan performed during an assisted fertility treatment, as most of the necessary information appears on the chart. The information I am particularly interested in is the following:]

- How many follicles have developed?
- What size they are?
- How many of them are mature on the day of the egg collection?
- How many of them are smaller and what sizes they are?
- How thick is the endometrium?
- How many eggs are fertilized?

- How many of them have become blastocysts?
- Were you prescribed Claxine, Aspirin for blood clotting, or steroids for NK cells?

[When patients come with this information, discussion can begin immediately. In fact, most unsuccessful IVF cases are due to the follicles not being mature enough; they are instead many different sizes as the ovaries are not fully functioning and are not responding fully to the drug stimulation.]

Recent blood test results
Have you had the following blood tests within the last six months?
Rubella antibodies (IgG)
Hepatitis B surface antigen
HIV antibody/antigen
Hepatitis C antibody
Chlamydia
Smear test

If yes, try to obtain a copy of the report prior to your initial consultation.

[If you have a lot of information, it would be even better if you sent it all to the clinic in advance. If possible, the doctor will look through all the information before your visit so you can spend your initial consultation discussing your situation rather than simply writing up your case notes.

If you have not had many tests, don't worry – this is what the fertility doctor is there for. Any tests you need can be arranged.]

What may be involved during a follow-up consultation

The purpose of a follow-up consultation is to analyse the effectiveness of the TCM treatment to date. Each time a patient turns up for a follow-up consultation, we look first at their temperature chart (see pages 70–73) to see how the ovaries are functioning and whether or not there is an improvement. I then ask general questions. The answers identify whether the woman's body, particularly the ovary, is in good form or whether something is out of balance.

The questions might include the following:

How has your sleeping been?

If a person sleeps well, their body and spirit is in balance.

If a person feels they can't get off to sleep, there could be some Liver Heat present.

If a person wakes up early or has to visit the bathroom in the night, that could indicate an obstruction in the abdominal environment, pressurizing the bladder.

Other people wake up early for psychological reasons, because they are worried about something.

How are your bowel movements?

If a person has loose bowel movements – diarrhoea several times a day – then I would look into whether they have a weak Stomach or whether their Spleen needs to improve. In some cases the problem may be due to Irritable Bowel Syndrome (IBS), which means there is inner tension.

If a person complains of constipation, it may be due to excessive Heat, which depletes fluids in the body.

Are you thirsty?

People can't usually tell whether they are thirsty, but if the immediate reply is, '*No, I am not thirsty,*' it means they don't really have a lot of Heat in the body.

If somebody says, '*I am really thirsty,*' then I would need to find out whether the person has a lot of Heat in the body.

The state of a person's tongue (see pages 32–33) and pulse (see page 33) help me to assess their answers. I consider what kind of tongue they have. Is it:

- Really dry?
- Really red?
- Very moist with a lot of coating?

I then look at their pulse. If someone says they are very thirsty, and the pulse is very fast and powerful, it means that they have an excess of Heat and too much *yang* in the body. The treatment will need to reduce the Heat to promote *yin*. On the other hand, if someone says they are very thirsty, but the pulse is not very strong and the tongue has no coating, there could be a *yin* deficiency. Then the treatment will need to build up the *yin* to promote body fluids.

It may be easy to reduce the Heat, but it will take a long time to build up the *yin*. It is rather like a running tap. When there is a lot of water, it is simple to draw some off. However, when the tap is blocked and water only drips out, you have to wait for it to accumulate, drop by drop. It is a much slower process.

SIGNS THAT YOUR BODY IS IN A HEALTHY CONDITION FOR CONCEPTION

1. **You are sleeping well** That is, falling asleep without difficulty and sleeping soundly. A normal sleep pattern should consistent of seven to eight hours a night. Good-quality sleep provides time for the body to restore its energy, ready for the next day. Sleeping too much, very deep sleep and needing long hours of sleep normally indicates that a person has Damp and Phlegm, which becomes heavily stagnant during sleep.

2. **You have a good pulse** In TCM terms the pulse would be described as slippery. 'Normal' slippery would indicate that the flow of energy is good but not 'aggressive'. 'Wiry' slippery is very tight and 'twangy', like a guitar. A wiry pulse may also be normal but can also sometimes be aggressive, which could indicate Liver stress.

3. **Your temperature chart is good** If it conforms to the standard pattern, it means the ovaries are in good form. See page 71 for a very good temperature chart. When a woman's body is in good form and the ovaries function well, the chart will look like this. If she has achieved three or more good cycles, then she is likely to be ready to conceive and the pregnancy is likely to happen in the near future. If the pattern is erratic, that means the cycle has not stabilized and the woman is not yet ready to conceive.

GLOSSARY

Acupuncture A treatment used in TCM. Fine needles are inserted into specific points of the body to help promote and balance the body's system.

Adhesion Body tissues, such as scar tissue, that have grown together but should be separated surgically.

Amenorrhea The absence of menstrual periods.

Anti-Mullerian hormone Thought to be a useful hormone marker for predicting ovarian reserve, ovarian ageing, ovarian dysfunction and ovarian responsiveness.

Antioxidant A substance that inhibits the destructive effects of oxidization. Maintaining a sufficient intake of antioxidants by eating the recommended five portions of fruit and vegetables each day will allow the body to compensate for free radicals. These highly reactive chemicals attack molecules and can damage sperm and eggs.

Antisperm antibodies Produced by the body's immune system, they cause sperm to bunch together, thus affecting their ability to reach and fertilize an egg.

Assisted fertility treatment When natural conception has not been possible, assisted conception methods such as ovulation induction, IVF, ICSI or IUI are undertaken.

Asthenozoospermia Reduced sperm motility.

Azoospermia The absence of live sperm in the seminal fluid.

BBT (Basal Body Temperature) (See pages 67–70.)

Blood deficiency Insufficient supply or quality of Blood in the body.

Blood stagnation When Blood circulation is unable to flow smoothly it becomes obstructed and stagnates in one area, which can lead to a functional disorder.

BMI Body Mass Index is a height versus weight calculation of body fat and is a useful tool to calculate your optimum weight.

Body fluids There are two different types of substances present in the body: *jin*, the lighter substance, which nourishes the skin and muscles; and *ye* a heavier substance which nourishes the brain, bone marrow, spine, joints and different sensory organs.

Chlamydia An often asymptomatic sexually transmitted disease caused by an organism, which may reduce the quality of sperm in a male and lead to severe pelvic inflammation in the female, which can damage the fallopian tubes.

Clinical pregnancy When there is an increasing level of HCG (human chorionic gonadotropin) or when an ultrasound scan shows that the gestational sac is within the uterus.

Conception The successful fertilization of a woman's egg by a man's sperm.

Contraceptive pill An oral medication for women used as a form of birth control. In some cases, when this hormonal method of contraception is stopped, periods do not return or become irregular, although for the majority of women their cycle returns to normal.

Corpus luteum The structure into which a follicle turns after ovulation. Its role is to produce hormones, such as progesterone.

Damp Excessive fluid retained in the body as a result of a digestion system malfunction.

Depression Couples who are having trouble conceiving, understandably, often experience feelings of sadness and despair, which can lead to depression. There is a healthy way to try to combat these low moods, including a healthy diet, rest and relaxation, and regular exercise.

Detox Removing or clearing out toxins in the body, thereby preventing disease.

DNA Sperm Fragmentation Test This test is thought to provide a reliable analysis of sperm DNA integrity, which semen analysis cannot always detect. It may help to identify men who are at risk of failing to initiate a healthy ongoing pregnancy.

Donor eggs In cases where a woman's eggs are of poor quality or low in quantity, donor eggs are a solution, and can significantly increase the chances of a pregnancy occurring.

Ectopic pregnancy A pregnancy that has implanted outside a woman's uterus, usually in the fallopian tube.

Egg (oocyte) The female reproductive cell produced by the ovary.

Egg collection The process of collecting a woman's unfertilized eggs to be artificially fertilized by procedures such as IVF or ICSI.

Embryo The fertilized ovum (egg).

Embryo transfer (ET) During assisted fertility treatment, a patient's embryos are cultured in a laboratory until they are of a satisfactory grade to be transferred back to the womb.

Endometriosis A condition in which cells from the lining of the uterus (womb) grow outside the uterus.

Endometrium The inner lining of the uterine wall; the structure, thickness and the state of the endometrium change during the menstrual cycle.

Fallopian tubes These two tubes lead from a woman's ovaries to the uterus, and are the place where the sperm usually fertilizes the egg during conception.

Fertilization The union of the woman's egg with the man's sperm, which results in an embryo.

Fibroid A benign (not cancerous) muscle growth in or around the uterus.

Fluctuating hormone levels Regular hormone level tests are important to assess the female reproductive system as hormones that fluctuate outside their normal range can lead to fertility problems.

Folic acid This supplement is recommended to women trying for a baby to help prevent spinal defects such as spina bifida. It should be taken every day up to the first three months of pregnancy.

Follicle A cell structure within the ovary that may contain an egg.

Frozen Embryo Transfer (FET) The replacement of embryos into the women's body that may have been previously frozen.

FSH (follicle stimulating hormone) A hormone that stimulates the growth of a mature egg in the ovaries and the production of sperm in the testes.

HCG (human chorionic gonadotropin) (See page 66.)

Hormone tests Regular hormone level checks are carried out as a matter of routine to monitor patients' progress. It is important to check that fertility hormones are within the normal range to ensure ovulation and conception. All blood tests, including FSH, LH, prolactin, oestradiol, Anti-Mullerian hormone and inhibin B can be easily organised through a laboratory.

HSG (hysterosalpingogram) An x-ray of the uterus and fallopian tubes taken after injection through the cervix of a radio-opaque dye. This is a routine procedure to check the structure of the fallopian tubes and the womb.

Hydrosalpinx A fallopian tube that is blocked at its outer end and filled with serous or clear fluid.

Hysteroscopy The inspection of the uterine cavity by endoscopy with access through the cervix.

ICSI (Intra-cytoplasmic Sperm Injection) A micro-manipulation technique where a single sperm is directly inserted into an individual egg. This procedure has a high rate of miscarriage, premature birth and chromosome abnormality. It is used with patients who have poor egg or sperm quality (particularly fewer sperm).

Implantation An early pregnancy event where the embryo adheres to the lining of the uterus.

Inhibin B One of the hormone markers that can be used to predict ovarian reserve, ovarian ageing, ovarian dysfunction and ovarian responsiveness.

Insemination To inject seminal fluid into the vagina, cervix or uterus.

IUI (Intra-Uterine Insemination) An assisted conception procedure, which does not involve egg retrieval and uses low doses of drugs to induce ovulation. The patient has an ultrasound scan to establish the number of follicles and their sizes and may use an HCG to ensure the eggs are released. The sperm is then washed and cleaned of bacteria by the laboratory and is inserted directly into the womb through the cervix.

IVF (In-Vitro Fertilization) An assisted conception procedure, which is considered for couples suffering from unexplained infertility, blocked or damaged fallopian tubes and male problems such as low sperm count or low motility. The eggs are surgically retrieved from the woman and fertilized with the man's washed sperm in a laboratory. The fertilized eggs are then introduced back to the womb for implantation.

Jing The basic constitution, nutritive essence, reproductive essence, seed.

Kidney function In TCM, this organ plays a major role in the urinary and reproductive systems, as well as in parts of the endocrine and nervous systems, more specifically egg and sperm production.

Laparoscopy The inspection of the ovaries, uterus and fallopian tubes by means of a laparoscope inserted through the abdominal wall.

LH (Luteinizing hormone) A hormone that regulates ovulation and menstruation in women, and in men stimulates testosterone production.

Liver function In TCM, this governs the free, uninterrupted flow of vital energy within the human body, which has a great influence over the menstrual cycle in women and is responsible for promoting a well-balanced circulation of qi in the body. It is believed to play a very important part in assisting successful ovulation and consequently conception.

Luteal phase The second half of the menstrual cycle, usually lasting 14 days, which starts after ovulation when the corpus luteum secretes large amounts of progesterone and ends with the beginning of the menstrual flow.

Male factor (male infertility) A term used when infertility is caused by problems for the male partner, such as low quantity and low quality of sperm.

Meridians The meridians in which energy flows around the body.

Miscarriage The natural loss of a pregnancy occurring any time between conception and 24 weeks of pregnancy. Also referred to as spontaneous abortion, it is the most common complication of early pregnancy.

Natural cycle of IVF The procedure of In-Vitro Fertilization carried out during a normal monthly cycle which therefore does not use powerful drugs to stimulate a woman's ovaries.

Natural killer cells (NK cells) White blood cells which some believe can overreact to a potential pregnancy, attacking the embryo and causing miscarriage. An immunology test can be performed in the case of implantation failure and recurrent miscarriage. This is an area of active research and the idea is still controversial.

Oestradiol The strongest naturally occurring form of oestrogen.

Oestrogen The female hormone produced by the follicles in the ovaries and responsible for ovulation.

Oligoasthenoteratozoospermia A very low sperm count, motility and elevated morphology.

Oligoasthenozoospermia A very low sperm count and motility.

Oocyte An immature ovum or egg cell that is produced in the ovary.

Organ A complete and independent part of the human body that has a specific function.

Ovarian reserve test A hormone test which measures levels of FSH, LH, oestradiol, prolactin, Anti-Mullerian hormone and inhibin B on Days 2 to 4 of a woman's menstrual cycle.

Ovaries Ovum-producing productive organs located in a woman's pelvis.

Ovulation The spontaneous release of a mature egg from an ovarian follicle.

Ovulation induction Stimulation of the ovaries by drugs in order to encourage the development of multiple follicles and therefore multiple eggs.

PCOS (Polycystic Ovary Syndrome)
A condition that causes the ovaries to overproduce male hormones due to a hormonal imbalance. This can prevent the normal growth of the egg follicles, causing multiple small cysts to form and resulting in the enlargement of the ovaries.

Pelvic Inflammatory Disease (PID)
An infection (generally bacterial) of the female pelvic organs, which originates in the vagina and works its way through to the womb and on to the fallopian tubes. This condition can sometimes affect the ovaries and, if left untreated, can cause the tubes to become blocked.

Peri-menopause The time in a woman's life just before menopause when her body starts making less oestrogen and progesterone (female hormones) and her chances of becoming pregnant are reduced.

PGS (Pre-implantation Genetic Screening) Early-stage genetic testing to identify chromosomal abnormalities in embryos.

Pituitary Gland A small gland, situated beneath the brain, with many functions, one of which is to secrete hormones such as FSH, which control ovulation.

Primary infertility The body's inability to produce a child.

Progesterone A hormone secreted by the corpus luteum after ovulation has occurred to prepare the uterus for implantation of the fertilized egg. It is vital in maintaining a pregnancy, particularly in the early stages, and in promoting development of the mammary glands.

Prolactin A hormone produced by the pituitary gland, which helps prepare breast milk during pregnancy.

Qi (pronounced 'chi') In TCM, vital energy that helps the Blood to flow.

Qi stagnation In TCM, when the vital energy stops flowing or moving.

Recurrent miscarriage A case of repeated miscarriages, which can be caused by factors such as foetal, placental or maternal abnormalities and is defined by a couple having had three or more miscarriages before 20 weeks gestation.

Secondary infertility A couple who have conceived in the past, whether resulting in a healthy live birth or miscarriage, who are now experiencing difficulties in conceiving again.

Semen Also referred to as seminal fluid, the discharge of the male ejaculation containing spermatozoa. This organic fluid, secreted by the male reproductive organs, fertilizes the female egg.

Semen analysis A test performed as part of regular baseline investigations for infertility, semen analysis reports on specific characteristics of a man's semen and the sperm contained within it. Important factors such as count, motility, volume and abnormal form play an important part in determining the quality of the sample.

Sperm (spermatozoa) The male reproductive cells contained in semen, which fertilize the egg during conception.

Sperm count (or sperm density) The total number of sperm per millilitre in the ejaculate.

Sperm morphology The shape of the sperm cells, in particular whether there are defects in the head, neck, midpiece or tail.

Sperm motility The sperm's ability to move towards the egg for fertilization. This is an important factor in the assessment of sperm quality.

TCM (Traditional Chinese Medicine) One of the oldest medical systems to be practised in the world, originally from China.

Testes The male reproductive glands, which are responsible for producing sperm and testosterone.

Thyroid A gland found in the neck responsible for producing the hormone thyroxin. An underactive or overactive thyroid producing insufficient or excessive amounts of thyroxin can affect other hormones in the body, which in turn can prevent ovulation or cause irregular periods.

Tubal patency test A baseline fertility investigation that determines whether the fallopian tubes are open and is used to detect whether there are any abnormalities delaying conception. (*See also Hysterosalpingogram*)

Ultrasound A non-invasive diagnostic radiology technique that uses ultrasonic waves instead of radiation to visualize internal body structures. It is also regularly used to monitor a developing foetus.

Unexplained infertility When no mechanical reason can be found for a couple's infertility, despite extensive investigations.

FURTHER RESOURCES

For further information about TCM and its role in fertility treatment contact The Zhai Clinic:

The Zhai Clinic
128 Harley Street
London W1G 7JT

Tel: +44 (0)20 7486 8438
Fax: +44 (0)20 7935 3510
Email: info@zhaiclinic.com
www.zhaiclinic.com

For more information on supplements from Dr Zhai, visit: www.zhaihealthcare.co.uk

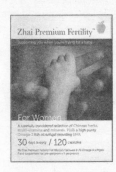 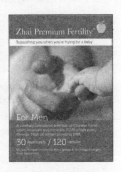

For further information about TCM, and to find a practitioner near you, contact:

The Association of Traditional Chinese
Medicine and Acupuncture, UK
5 Grosvenor House
1 High Street
Edgware
London HA8 7TA

Tel: +44 (0)20 8951 3030
Fax: +44 (0)20 8951 3030
Email: info@atcm.co.uk
www.atcm.co.uk

INDEX

Major page references are in **bold**; illustrations are in *italics*.
Herbal formulas are indicated by (H) following the name.

P

pak choi
  lightly boiled pak choi 216
palpitations 27, 109, 156
  acupressure points 227
Pelvic Inflammatory Disease (PID) 80, **95**, 103, 128, 266
Pelvic Inflammatory Disease (PID)
  and Damp-Heat 147
  herbal formulas 174
Penetrating Vessel 51, **52**, 104, 107, 108, 109, 137, 138, 151, 156
  see also uterus
penis
  yellow discharge 111
  see also erectile dysfunction
Pensiveness 31
peri-menopause 90, 122, 159, 265
  and Blood Heat 151
  case study 109–110, 162–164
Pericardium 27, 29, 48
  meridian 47, 229
periods 17
  acupressure points 226, 227, 228
  clotting 21
  herbal formulas 173–174, **177–178**
  irregular 26, 137
  irregular (case study) 64
  lack of 109
  late starting 108
  and menstrual cycle 64–67
  and moxibustion 233
  painful 21, 106, 148, 226, 227
personality 142
  see also shen
Phlegm-Damp 106
  acupressure points 228
  case study 126, 147
  diet for 209–210
  herbal formulas 182
  questions to determine type 125–126
  symptoms 144–145
  treatment 145–146
Phlegm-Heat 105

physical activity, excessive 103
physical inspection 32
pills 169
pinellia root 186
pituitary gland 65, **90**, 266
  and acupuncture 38
placenta 235
polycystic ovaries 57, 60, 72
  and Blood and qi deficiency 155
  and Blood deficiency 109
  and Blood stasis 137
  case study 73–75, 76–77
  and Cold in the uterus 153–154
  and Dampness 104
  diet 204
  and Phlegm-Damp 144
Polycystic Ovary Syndrome (PCOS) 91–92, 265
  case study 92–93, 147, 167–168
  diet 204
  and Kidney yang deficiency 166
polyps 95
polyunsaturated fats 193–194
porridge 214
post partum bleeding, herbal formulas 183
postnatal qi 20
powder 170
pre-eclampsia 248–249
pre-heaven essence 107
Pre-implantation Genetic Diagnosis (PGD) 17
Pre-implantation Genetic Screening (PGS) 266
pregnancy
  and acupressure 225
  and age 56, 63, **90**, **159**
  biochemical 75
  bleeding during 27, 172–173
  breech 234
  clinical 261–262
  ectopic 95, 137, 140, 147, 173–174, 262
  first trimester 235–238
  food cravings 235
  herbal formulas 237
  herbs to avoid 187–188
  herbs to support 186–188
  high blood pressure 28, 245–246, 248–249

Regulate the period tea 157, **177–178**
relaxation, acupressure points 232
reproductive essence (*jing*) 28
reproductive health 8–9
restlessness 27
Restore the right Kidney pill 185
retrograde ejaculation 100
rooibos (red bush) tea 207

S
sadness 28
salty foods 205
San Bao **22–24**
saturated fats 194–195
scutellaria 187
second trimester 238–239
secondary infertility 64, 266
selenium 198
self-prescription 117, **171**
semen 266
  analysis 83–85, 256, 266
seminal fluid 112
senses, five 27
Seven Emotions 31
sexual intercourse 69, 70
sexually transmitted diseases 80, 93, 95, 103
shen 22, 24
Six Excesses 30–31
Six flavour tea 161, **176–177**
skin, dry 109, 155, 159, 160
sleep problems in pregnancy 249
Small Intestine 25–26, 29, 43
  foods for 205
  meridian 44
Smaller Meridians 51–52
smelling 32
smoking 203, 219
Sorrow 31
soup
  Ping's chicken soup 216
sour foods 205
sperm 266
  abnormal 17
  absence of in semen 99

and acupuncture 38
count 17, 38, 84, 85–86, **98–99**, 111, 112,
  161, 266
count (case study) 97–98
density 267
DNA fragmentation 84, 262
ICSI (Intra-Cytoplasmic Sperm Injection)
  57, 58
and Kidney *yang* deficiency 166
morphology 267
motility 17, 38, **84–85**, 86, **99**, 111, 267
quality of 10–11, 13, 29, 38, **99**
test results 99
spirit 24
  see also shen
Spleen 25–26, **28–29**, 42, 103
  acupressure points 227
  and Blood deficiency 109
  and Dampness 104–105
  foods for 205
  herbal formulas 174–176, 178
  meridian 42, 227
  see also qi
Spleen *qi* 20, 133
Spleen *qi* deficiency 103
  herbal formulas 175
spotting 68
  and Blood stasis 137
  case study 76–77
stagnation
  of Blood 21
  of *qi* 21
stickiness and Phlegm-Damp 145
stillbirth 153–154
stimulating foods 206–207
stir-fried beef with egg and tomato 217
stir-fried chicken with vegetables 218
Stomach 25–26, 30
  acupressure points 226, 227
  bloated 105
  foods for 205
  meridian 41, 226–227
  see also qi
Stomach *qi* and pregnancy 237

stools
    blood in 144
    dry 160
    loose 104, 148, 165
    and Phlegm-Damp 145
    sticky 144, 145
    see also diarrhoea
stress 219
    acupressure points 228, 229
    herbal formulas 174–176
    see also anxiety
sugar cravings 202
surgical intervention 11, 29, 87, 118
    Blood stasis type 137
    and Damp-Heat 148
    and infertility **103**
sweet foods 205
swelling 27, 125
    in pregnancy 248
    see also oedema
Szechuan lovage root 186

T
Tai Chi 222
Tao Hong Si Wu Tang (H) **181**
Tea to reinforce yin 161, **178–180**
teas 170, 210
    healing properties of 207–208
temper, short 28
temperature, taking 71–72
testes 267
testicles
    acupressure points 227
    keeping cool 219
    lumps and swelling 100
    problems with 99–100
    undescended 100
testicular cancer 100
testicular failure 99
testosterone
    low levels (men) 100
    raised levels (women) 91–92
thermometers 69, 71–72
Three Treasures 22–24

throat, dry 159–160
thrush 128
thyroid 92, 160, 165, 267
Tiao Jing Tang (H) 157, **177–178**
tinnitus 159
    acupressure points 229
tiredness 104, 145
    acupressure points 226, 228
    in pregnancy 243
tongue **32–33**, 33
    and Blood stasis 137
    bluish-purple 153
    colour 32–33
    crimson 137
    diagnosis 32–33
    pale 109, 153, 155, 165
    pale and sticky 104
    pale and wet 109
    pink 141, 155
    purple 21, 32–33, 105
    purple spots 137
    and qi stagnation 105
    red 108, 151
    red (men) 111, 112
    sticky 104
    swollen 104, 165
    veins underneath 137
    wet 109, 165
tongue, coating 33
    greasy 145, 148
    greasy (men) 111
    none 160
    thick white 154
    thin 141
    wet 153
    yellow 148
tonifying 116
toxicity, reducing 22
Traditional Chinese Medicine (TCM) 8–9, 267
    approach to diagnosis 20, 88
    approach to treatment 13, 18, 20, 22,
        114–115
    benefits of 59–60
    combined with IVF 57

ACKNOWLEDGEMENTS

AUTHOR'S ACKNOWLEDGEMENTS

This book would not have been written without all the encouragement and tremendous support I have received. I have many people to thank for helping me on my journey to publication. I have been extremely fortunate to have Denise Bates as my publisher and Clare Hulton as my agent. From the moment they first approached me I knew I would have to look no further to find the ideal people to represent and publish my book. Their excellence and professionalism has been evident every step of the way. I am grateful, too, to Sally Morris, Joanna Smith, Jo Murray and Leanne Bryan, the talented editors who helped to shape the words and place the material on the right pages and in a readable order; and to the rest of the team at Octopus books for their commitment and enthusiasm for this project. I would also like to thank my dedicated and skilful team at the Zhai Clinic, especially Toni Maughan and Jane Godoy, for their professional assistance – and my wonderful patients, past and present, for sharing their stories with me. Mr Stuart Lavery and Mr Michael Dooley deserve a special mention for embracing TCM as a discipline and for endorsing my work. It is a great pleasure to work in collaboration with them; special thanks to Sarah Sutton for her patience and hard work and for taking all the pressure away from me. Finally I would like to thank John, for his unerring care and support.

Dr Xiao-Ping Zhai

PUBLISHER'S ACKNOWLEDGEMENTS

Senior Editor Leanne Bryan
Copy Editor Joanna Smith
Executive Art Editor Jonathan Christie
Designer www.theoakstudo.co.uk
Illustrator Abi Read
Picture Researcher Giulia Hetherington
Senior Production Controller Lucy Carter

PICTURE CREDITS

Pictures are listed in page order.
18 Hemera/Thinkstock; 68, 89a and b Grei/Shutterstock; 98 Dorling Kindersley